Praise for
Every Man's Battle

"Every male should read this book. As the battle for our minds intensifies, the need for direction increases. This book offers timely and timeless counsel."
—MAX LUCADO, pastor and best-selling author

"Sexual temptation is more prevalent than ever before, hounding men in every moment of every day, through our phones, movies, TV, the internet, and more. Stephen Arterburn and Fred Stoeker recognized the growing need to shift the conversation, and they put forth a resource to help men overcome their struggles and achieve victory. Countless lives and marriages have been transformed already by the principles in *Every Man's Battle,* and this thoroughly updated guide to living with integrity will propel that impact even farther."
—JOSH D. McDOWELL, author and speaker

"There is no more common enemy of true manhood than the diversion or the perversion of our sexual capacities. I welcome every contribution to the arsenal of resistance."
—JACK W. HAYFORD, LittD, former pastor of the Church on the Way
and founder and chancellor of the King's Seminary

"This book will revolutionize the marriage of every man who reads it. Why? Because every man battles sexual temptations, and every marriage grows stronger when these temptations are defeated. The vulnerable, honest, and insightful pages of this book reveal what every man must know."
—DRS. LES AND LESLIE PARROTT, authors of *Saving Your Marriage Before It Starts*

"This timely resource presents clear, practical principles for sexual purity. Arterburn and Stoeker call for courage, commitment, and self-discipline as they lead men into a more successful relationship with God, family, and spouse. This book is truly for every man."
—DR. JOHN C. MAXWELL, founder of the INJOY Group

"God has used Steve Arterburn countless times to impact my heart and life; I am thankful for him and his investment in *Every Man's Battle*. I am also grateful for Fred Stoeker. Fred pours himself into this book with honesty, vulnerability, and a practical strategy to fight the good fight. He offers biblical truth and hope to anyone with ears to hear how to battle the war of sexual temptation. Read with an open heart, *Every Man's Battle* may save your marriage and your witness."

—DR. GARY ROSBERG, president of America's Family Coaches

"Having grown up in a machismo world and getting caught up in gangs before I turned to the Lord in prison, I definitely needed to read *Every Man's Battle* when it came out twenty years ago—and I'm glad I did."

—CASEY DIAZ, author of *The Shot Caller*

Every Man's Battle

Revised and Updated 20th Anniversary Edition

Every Man's Battle

Winning the War on Sexual Temptation
One Victory at a Time

WORKBOOK INCLUDED

Stephen Arterburn
Fred Stoeker
with Mike Yorkey

WATERBROOK

Every Man's Battle, Revised and Updated 20th Anniversary Edition

All Scripture quotations, unless otherwise indicated, are taken from the Holy Bible, New International Version®, NIV®. Copyright © 1973, 1978, 1984, 2011 by Biblica Inc.® Used by permission. All rights reserved worldwide. Scripture quotations marked (AMP) are taken from the Amplified Bible. Copyright © 2015 by the Lockman Foundation. Used by permission. (www.Lockman.org). Scripture quotations marked (KJV) are taken from the King James Version.

Italics in Scripture quotations reflect the author's added emphasis.

Details in some anecdotes and stories have been changed to protect the identities of the persons involved.

The information on sexual addiction in chapter 3 is drawn from Stephen Arterburn's *Addicted to "Love"* (Ann Arbor, MI: Vine, 1991), 109–10.

Trade Paperback ISBN 978-0-525-65351-6
eBook ISBN 978-0-593-19272-6

Every Man's Battle copyright © 2000, 2020 by Stephen Arterburn, Fred Stoeker, and Mike Yorkey
Every Man's Battle Workbook copyright © 2002, 2020 by Stephen Arterburn, Fred Stoeker, and Mike Yorkey

Cover design by Mark D. Ford

The authors are represented by Alive Literary Agency, www.aliveliterary.com.

Published in the United States by WaterBrook, an imprint of Random House, a division of Penguin Random House LLC.

WATERBROOK® and its deer colophon are registered trademarks of Penguin Random House LLC.

Library of Congress Cataloging-in-Publication Data
Names: Arterburn, Stephen, 1953– author. | Stoeker, Fred, author. | Yorkey, Mike, author.
Title: Every man's battle : winning the war on sexual temptation one victory at a time / Stephen Arterburn and Fred Stoeker, with Mike Yorkey.
Description: Revised and Updated 20th Anniversary Edition. | Colorado Springs : WaterBrook, 2020. | Includes bibliographical references.
Identifiers: LCCN 2019019872 | ISBN 9780525653516 (pbk.) | ISBN 9780593192726 (electronic)
Subjects: LCSH: Sex—Religious aspects—Christianity. | Temptation. | Christian men—Religious life.
Classification: LCC BT708 .A77 2020 | DDC 241/.664—dc23
LC record available at https://lccn.loc.gov/2019019872

Printed in the United States of America
2020—Revised Edition

7th Printing

SPECIAL SALES
Most WaterBrook books are available at special quantity discounts when purchased in bulk by corporations, organizations, and special-interest groups. Custom imprinting or excerpting can also be done to fit special needs. For information, please email specialmarketscms@penguinrandomhouse.com.

From Stephen Arterburn

To my friend Jim Burns.
You have displayed great love
and been a premier example of sexual integrity.

From Fred Stoeker

To my heavenly Father (thank You that You ran to me);
to my wife, Brenda;
and to my friends Dave Johnson and Les Flanders.

Contents

Part V: Victory with Your Mind

Part VI: Victory in Your Heart

Part VII: Restoring Your Sexuality Together

Workbook

This book is often quite explicit in how the coauthors describe past struggles—their own and others'—with sexual purity. For the sake of communicating honestly with readers who face similar struggles, our goal has been to achieve frankness without causing offense, thereby making it easier for men to face up to any uncleanness and press forward by God's grace and power into actively sharing His holiness.

A Letter to Wives from Brenda Stoeker

While *Every Man's Battle* is directed primarily to married men, we highly recommend that every wife and serious girlfriend read it as well.

This book gives women a greater understanding of what men are up against as they battle the age-old problem of the eyes, since by nature women are nowhere near as visual in their sexuality and therefore don't understand this male battle from personal experience. That's important, because the truth is that male sexuality can be unsettling—even shocking—to women.

This vast difference in the sexual wiring between men and women often confounds wives. For instance, I once wrote the following in response to a survey that Fred gave me on the topic:

> I don't want to sound mean, but because women don't generally experience this sexual sin problem in the same way that men do, it can seem to us that men are uncontrolled perverts who don't think about anything but sex.

Strong words, but straight from this woman's heart. That's just how outrageous these differences can seem to us as wives, and when it comes to a husband's sexual sin, these differences in wiring create a natural tug-of-war in a wife's heart between pity and disgust for his situation, as well as a struggle between mercy and judgment.

What's a wife to do? Because of these differences, I strongly believe nothing is more important than to get educated about male sexuality. Maleness does matter, so we women need to understand it. Maleness isn't toxic or perverted; it's just different. And if we're to get past throwing stones and get on to building sexual relationships that are pleasing to God, we need to be reading and learning, listening and giving. Your husband needs you sexually, and as his wife, you are God's only answer to that need.

I'll be the first to admit I didn't always have the right attitude toward my husband on this topic. In our early years of marriage, I was stretched deeply by Fred's sexuality—especially by its visual orientation and its regular need for expression. Male sexuality seemed rather shallow and almost weird to me! But before long, I discovered that it really isn't shallow; it's just different. And given the obvious struggle men have with sexual purity when they go without sex, I began to understand why God would tell me, "Your body is not your own" (see 1 Corinthians 7:4). I learned that sex is vital not only to Fred's purity but also to his emotional intimacy with me.

That's not to say that a husband should have sex any time and every time he wants it! I'm simply saying that a husband's sexual purity is not just every man's battle but every *couple's* battle.

In this updated version, Steve and Fred address more recent developments in male sexual behavior, in particular the troubling disinterest of some husbands for sexual intimacy with their wives. Sadly, this puzzling reality is often connected to increasingly vulgar and intense pornography, which can cause the much-publicized erectile dysfunction (ED). Of course, a husband's ED may have a physical cause for which a physician's involvement is required, but the ED also may be the destructive result of the brain's rewiring. These topics are discussed in this edition of *Every Man's Battle,* and some ideas are offered on how to regain appropriate physical intimacy in your marriage.

I urge you to open your heart to the words that follow. Seize the day—for yourself, for your marriage, and for your family.

Introduction to the Updated and Revised Edition

From Steve Arterburn

When the publisher first called me in 1999 and I agreed to read Fred Stoeker's manuscript, unexpectedly I found myself stirred by a message that would impact the Christian world in amazing ways.

Fred's teaching was different. He did not shame the reader or minimize the problem. Best of all, he laid out a practical, easy-to-understand path to victory over a common plague infecting the character of Christian men everywhere. I was convinced that *Every Man's Battle* could transform more marriages more deeply than nearly any marriage book I could think of, and I wanted to be part of that.

How does a book on male sexual purity do this? Because it directly addresses the sexual sins that are the termites in the walls and foundations of just about every marriage today. On my phone-in *New Life Live!* radio broadcasts, we could easily do a one-hour show on pornography's chains every day of the week. In fact, we get so many calls from men desperate for freedom from impure thought lives and ungodly sexual actions that our screener has to limit those types of calls. I'm sure that even *more* men would phone in if they didn't feel so ashamed.

This is why I can confidently state that the book you now hold in your hands has the potential to free you from sexual sin and allow you to love your wife in ways you never dreamed possible. Why? Because the teaching and principles we share have done just that for millions of readers over the past twenty years. About a year after *Every Man's Battle* was first published, it was already a phenomenon. It became the most frequently reordered book in Christian bookstores with an endless line of pastors, men's ministry leaders, and past readers buying dozens of copies for their Bible studies, men's-group meetings, friends, and family members.

Of course, the impact on men's lives was immediate, and the ripple effects healed families, organizations, churches, and communities. A grassroots movement of support groups and study groups formed in church basements and college dorms. Thousands of men attended New Life's Every Man's Battle workshops. In retrospect, I can only shake my head in wonder and gratitude over being part of a project that has changed so many lives.

As of today, Fred and I have written and published six books together: *Every Man's Battle, Every Man's Marriage, Every Young Man's Battle, Preparing Your Son for Every Man's Battle, Every Man's Challenge,* and *Every Heart Restored.* The entire Every Man series—which also includes several related books for men and women and a series of workbooks and Bible studies to enhance the understanding of the reader—has sold over three million copies worldwide, and *Every Man's Battle* has been published in twenty-three languages.

So, here we stand, twenty years later, celebrating what God has done and publishing this twentieth-anniversary edition. As you read, remember that we've changed the names of people in this book and have even altered a few details of their stories to protect their identities. But their stories are real. They are stories of men from all walks of life: white-collar office workers and blue-collar employees, as well as pastors, worship leaders, deacons, and elders. All of them are caught in a terrible snare, just as we once were.

You're in a tough position. You live in a world awash with sensual images available twenty-four hours a day in a variety of mediums: print, television, video, the internet, and smartphones. But God offers you freedom from the slavery of sin through the Cross of Christ, and He created your eyes and mind with the ability to be trained and controlled. We simply have to stand up and walk by His power on the right path. To do this, we need a battle plan, and you'll have one when you finish reading *Every Man's Battle*—a detailed strategy for living in sexual integrity.

Fred and I write from the perspective of married men, but the practical defenses we share in this book also apply to teens, young-adult men, and divorced men who must deal with the issue of sexual integrity while single. We want to help keep single men of all ages from lusting or developing addictive behavior and instead increase their odds of marrying the right women.

Every Man's Battle will challenge you in many ways. But in facing and overcoming these hurdles, you will find a route to rewarding sexual integrity.

From Fred Stoeker

So, how did *Every Man's Battle* come about? The answer is simple: sexual immorality once held me captive, and after being liberated, I wanted to help other men get free.

After teaching on the topic of male sexual purity in Sunday school in the late 1980s, I was approached one day by a man who said, "I always thought that since I was a man, I would not be able to control my roving eyes. I didn't know it could be any other way. Now I'm free!" Conversations like that thrilled my heart and confirmed the desire God gave me to help other men out of this quagmire.

As men shared with me their stories of sexual sin, many asked me to write a book. At first I passed this off as simple complimentary talk. After all, anything I committed to paper had little chance of being published. I'd never written a book before, I wasn't the host of a national radio show, I didn't have a PhD, and I hadn't gone to seminary. So, why did I start writing a book? Because I felt deeply that if God would grant me such a voice in His kingdom, I could give even more men some practical steps toward victory and being set free to help others.

The following passage inspired me to keep plodding away on this book night after night, month after month:

> Have mercy on me, O God,
>   according to your unfailing love;
> according to your great compassion
>   blot out my transgressions.
> Wash away all my iniquity
>   and cleanse me from my sin. . . .
> Restore to me the joy of your salvation
>   and grant me a willing spirit, to sustain me.

Then I will teach transgressors your ways,

and that sinners will turn back to you. (Psalm 51:1–2, 12–13)

Get it? God's plan is to set sinners free and wash them up so they can teach others. God has been using me in just that way. Forty years ago, God made me His own and thoroughly cleansed me. Twenty years ago, He sent me out to teach others His ways through the release of *Every Man's Battle*. Today, and with this twentieth-anniversary edition, He continues turning men back to Him. His plan for you remains the same as it's always been for His sons: to purify you and then send you out on a great adventure to liberate others.

And we need you out there. Pornographers have grown more vile and more depraved in the last twenty years. Now shamelessly creating and streaming porn for women, they've managed to addict our sisters and daughters on a broad scale for the first time in history, even though their sexuality is not as visual as it is in men. Formerly reliable female authors and speakers have even lost their way in this blitzkrieg, shell shocked by depravity's blast. Instead of taking an aggressive stand against porn's corrupting influence, some have fallen prey to the lures of the industry. And, as if that's not enough, today's pornography for *men* is vastly more vicious and twisted, inflicting a dramatic deterioration in a guy's ability to perform sexually in the master bedroom. So, this edition includes an all-new part 7 to help explain how porn and masturbation may have ravaged your sexuality and degraded your ability to share genuine, interpersonal intimacy with each other, heart to heart—along with steps you can take to turn that situation around.

We've also updated *Every Man's Battle* with some of the critical advances in brain science made over the past two decades, explaining how these discoveries back up our original positions and strengthen your ability to apply the practical steps that we're sharing so that you might win this battle once and for all.

Are you eager to get started? Good . . . so am I! Today more than ever, we need men of honor and decency, with their hands where they belong, with their eyes and minds focused on Christ. If roving eyes or sexually impure thoughts or even sexual addiction are issues in your life, Steve and I want you to do something about it.

Isn't it time?

Part I

Where We Are

1

Our Stories

A mong you there must not be even a hint of sexual immorality, or of any kind of impurity" (Ephesians 5:3). If there's a single Bible verse that captures God's standard for sexual purity, this is it.

And it compels this question: *In relation to God's standard, is there even a hint of sexual impurity in my life?*

For both of us the answer to that question was yes.

From Steve: Collision

On a sun-splashed Southern California morning years ago, I hopped into my Mercedes 450SL, white with a black top. The classic coupe was over ten years old but was still the car of my dreams. I'd owned it for just two months, and on that spectacular morning, with the top down and the wind blowing in my face, I was feeling especially good about life and my future.

I was tooling northbound through Malibu on my way to Oxnard on the PCH, as locals called the Pacific Coast Highway. I'd always loved driving on these four lanes of blacktop that hugged the golden coastline and provided a close-up view of LA's beach culture.

I never intentionally set out to be girl watching that day, but I spotted her about two hundred yards ahead and to the left. She was jogging toward me along the coastal sidewalk. From my sheepskin-covered leather seat, I found the view outstanding, even by California's high standards.

My eyes locked on to this goddess-like blonde, rivulets of sweat cascading down her tanned body as she ran at a purposeful pace. Her jogging outfit, if it could be called that in those days before sports bras and spandex, was actually a skimpy bikini. As she approached on my left, two tiny triangles of tie-dyed fabric struggled to contain her ample bosom.

I can't tell you what her face looked like; nothing above the neckline registered with me that morning. My eyes feasted on this banquet of glistening flesh as she passed on my left, and they continued to follow her lithe figure as she continued jogging southbound. Simply by lustful instinct, as if mesmerized by her gait, I turned my head further and further, craning my neck to capture every possible moment for my mental video camera.

Then *blam!*

I might still be marveling at this remarkable specimen of female athleticism if my Mercedes hadn't plowed into a Chevy Chevelle that had come to a complete stop in my lane. Fortunately, I was traveling only fifteen miles per hour in the stop-and-go traffic, but the mini-collision crumpled my front bumper and crinkled the hood. And the fellow I smacked into didn't appreciate the considerable damage to his Chevy's rear end.

I got out of the car—embarrassed, humiliated, saturated with guilt, and unable to offer a satisfying explanation. No way would I tell this guy, "Well, if you'd seen what I saw, you'd understand."

Sadly, I was the one who didn't fully understand what I had done or what was going on inside me. I continued in that darkness for quite some time before realizing I needed to make dramatic changes in the way I looked at women and the way I was relating to God.

From Fred: Wall of Separation

It happened every Sunday morning during our church worship service. I'd look around and see other men with their eyes closed, freely and intensely worshipping the God of the universe. Myself? I sensed only a wall of separation between the Lord and me.

Somehow, I wasn't right with God. As a new Christian, I imagined I just didn't know God well enough yet and that I'd grow into that connection. But as time passed, nothing changed. When I mentioned to my wife, Brenda, that I felt vaguely unworthy of Him, she wasn't the least bit surprised.

"Well, of course you don't!" she exclaimed. "You've never felt worthy of your own father. Every preacher I've known says that a man's relationship with his earthly father tremendously impacts his relationship with his heavenly Father."

"You could be right," I allowed.

I hoped it was that simple. I mulled it over as I recalled my days of youth.

My father, handsome and tough, had been a national wrestling champion in college and a bulldog in business. Aching to be like him, I'd joined my middle school wrestling team. But the best wrestlers are natural-born killers, and I soon found that I didn't have a wrestler's heart.

At the time, my dad was coaching wrestling on an interim basis at a small high school in Alburnett, Iowa. Though I was still in middle school, he wanted me to wrestle with the older guys, so he brought me along to the high school workouts.

One afternoon we were practicing escapes, and my partner was in the down position. While grappling on the mat, he suddenly needed to blow his nose. He straightened up, pulled his T-shirt to his nose, and violently emptied the contents onto the front of his shirt. We quickly returned to wrestling. As the up man, I was supposed to keep a tight grip on him. Reaching around his belly, my hand slid into his slimy T-shirt. Sickened, I let him go.

Dad, seeing him escape so easily, dressed me down. "What kind of man are you?" he roared, and then he screamed on and on at me for what seemed like forever. Staring hard at the mat during this onslaught, I realized that if I had a wrestler's heart, I would have cranked down tightly and ridden out my opponent in spite of the snot on my hands, maybe grinding his face into the mat in retaliation. But I hadn't, and after two more hollow, joyless years on the mat, I finally hung up my singlet for good.

I still wanted to prove myself to Dad, of course, so I tried other sports, excelling at football and baseball. But my father never forgave me for quitting wrestling, and

I couldn't quite prove myself to him as a man no matter how well I played on the gridiron or baseball diamond. And he never let me forget it.

He was verbally relentless. After I struck out in one baseball game, I hung my head on the way back to the dugout. "Get your head up!" he hollered for all to hear. I was mortified. On the car ride home, he ripped me so hard that I threw up into my ball cap. One time after he'd dropped me off at home and returned to his own place across town (he was divorced from my mom at the time), he wrote me a long letter detailing every mistake I'd made that day and dropped it in the mail that night.

And you know what? I never did measure up as a man, at least not in *his* mind. Years later, after I'd married Brenda, my father felt she had too much say in our marriage. "Real men take charge of their households," he said.

The Monster

So now, as Brenda and I discussed my relationship with my dad, she suggested I might need counseling. "It surely couldn't hurt," she said.

So I read some books and counseled with my pastor, and my feelings toward Dad improved. Still, I continued to feel that distance from God during the Sunday morning worship services, which revealed that Brenda's hunch was incorrect. My poor relationship with my dad wasn't the main culprit after all.

The true reason for that distance slowly dawned on me over time: there was a hint of sexual immorality in my life. In fact, there was a monster lurking about, and it surfaced each Sunday morning when I settled into my comfy La-Z-Boy and opened the newspaper. I would quickly find the department-store inserts and begin paging through the colored newsprint filled with models posing in bras and panties. Always smiling. Always available. I loved lingering over each ad insert. I rationalized to myself, *It's wrong, but it's such a small thing! Besides, it's a far cry from* Playboy, *right? And haven't I already given that up?*

So every Sabbath, I peered through the panties, fantasizing. Inevitably, I'd masturbate while on the couch. Occasionally, a model reminded me of a girl I once knew, and my mind rekindled the memories of our times together. I rather enjoyed my Sunday mornings with the newspaper.

As I examined myself more closely, I found I had more than a hint of sexual immorality. Even my sense of humor reflected it. Sometimes a person's innocent phrase—even from our pastor—struck me with a double sexual meaning. I would chuckle, but I felt uneasy.

Why do these double entendres come to my mind so easily? Should a Christian mind create them so nimbly? I remembered that the Bible said that such things shouldn't even be mentioned among the saints. *I'm worse,* I thought. *I even laugh at them!*

And my eyes? They were ravenous heat seekers searching the horizon, locking on any target with sensual heat: young mothers in shorts leaning over to pull children out of car seats, church soloists with silky shirts, college girls in low-cut summer dresses.

My mind, too, ran wherever it willed. This had begun in my childhood, when I found *Playboy* magazines under Dad's bed. He also subscribed to *Sex to Sexty*, a publication filled with jokes and comic strips with sexual themes. When Dad divorced Mom and moved to his bachelor's pad, he hung a giant velvet nude in his living room, overlooking us as we played cards on my Sunday afternoon visits.

Dad gave me a list of chores around his place when I was there. Once, I came across a nude photo of his mistress. On another occasion, I found an eight-inch dildo, which he obviously used in his kinky sex games with his new playmate.

Hope for the Hopeless

All this sexual stuff churned deep inside me, destroying a purity that wouldn't return for many years. Settling into college at Stanford University, I soon found myself drowning in pornography. I actually memorized the dates when my favorite soft-core porn magazines arrived at the local drugstore so in those pre-internet days I could get my hands on the new pictures as quickly as possible each month. I especially loved the "Girls Next Door" section of *Gallery* magazine, featuring pictures of nude girls taken by their boyfriends and submitted to the magazine.

Far from home in Iowa and without any Christian underpinnings, I descended by small steps into a sexual pit. The first time I had sexual intercourse, I just *knew* it was with a girl I would marry. The next time, it was with a girl I *thought* I would marry. The time after that, it was with a good friend that I might learn to love. Then it was with a female I barely knew who simply wanted to see what sex was like before graduating from Stanford. Eventually, I had sex with any girl at any time.

After several years in California, I found myself with four "steady" girlfriends simultaneously. I was sleeping with three of them and was essentially engaged to marry two of them. None knew of the others.

Why do I share all this?

First, so you'll know that I understand what it's like to be sexually ensnared in a deep pit. Second, I want to provide you with hope. As you'll soon see, God worked with me and lifted me out of that pit.

If there's even a hint of sexual immorality in your life, He will work with you as well.

2

Paying the Price

From Fred: Knowing Whom to Call

Despite the deepening, reeking sexual pigsty I occupied in my single days living in the Bay Area, I didn't notice anything wrong with my life. I was in college, for heaven's sake! I was only doing what college guys do, right? *Nothing wrong with that.*

Oh, sure, I attended church sporadically, and from time to time the pastor's words penetrated my heart and stirred up a bit of silt and guilt. But who was *he*? Besides, I loved my girlfriends, and they loved me. *No one's getting hurt,* I reasoned.

But God possessed a different line of reasoning, and He intended to be heard on this matter. My dad had eventually remarried, but as he skipped along matrimony's way, he hadn't invited just a new wife into his heart. He'd asked Jesus Christ in, to boot, and now whenever I visited back home in Iowa during college breaks, my dad and stepmother would drag me across the Mississippi River to the Moline Gospel Temple in Moline, Illinois. The gospel was clearly preached there, but to me the whole scene was ludicrous. I often laughed cynically. Those people were crazy!

On the surface, this young, proud intellectual appeared bulletproof to the truth. But beneath it all lay a closely held secret: an extreme, bone-crushing loneliness was devouring my soul.

Lonely? But, Fred, didn't you have four girlfriends?

I know. I was baffled too. I'd always heard that the best way to get to know a girl was to sleep with her, but the more girlfriends I added to my life and my bedroom, the more desperate and disconnected I became.

I'd been misinformed. The truth is, having early sex is the quickest way to wreck a budding relationship. So now, like a gerbil on his wheel, I rode a relentless spin to nowhere. Desperation gripped my very soul. God had me right where He wanted me.

After graduating from Stanford University with an honors degree in sociology, I decided to take a job in the San Francisco area as an investment advisor. One evening, I stayed late at the office to make a handful of evening telephone calls. When I looked up from my phone a bit later, I noticed that everyone else had gone home, leaving me alone with some troubling thoughts. As I cleaned up my desk before heading home for the night, I glanced out the window and was struck by the lovely burst of colors arching across the dusky sky. Immediately, I swiveled my chair around and propped my feet on the credenza to gaze into a typically grand California sunset.

I still don't know how God did it that evening, but all at once the colors faded from my attention. As the sun dipped beneath the horizon, I suddenly saw in full clarity what I had become, especially in regard to women. While I'd once been blind, now I could see, and what I saw was hopelessly ugly. Instantly, I saw my deep, deep need for a Savior. Gratefully, because of the Moline Gospel Temple, I knew whom to call upon.

My prayer that twilight evening was simple: "Lord, I'm ready to work with You if You're ready to work with me." I stood up and walked out of the office, not yet fully realizing what I'd just done. But God knew, and it seemed as if all heaven moved into my life. Within two weeks I had a job back in Iowa and a new life ahead of me. And no girlfriends!

Feeling Good

Once settled in Des Moines, I began attending a marriage class led by Joel Budd, the associate pastor of my new church. You might wonder why a single guy without a girlfriend would ever attend a marriage class. The answer was simple to me: I knew full well that if there was anything that God needed to teach me, it was how to treat women properly. So when I visited that church for the first time and saw the list of Sunday school classes, I knew that the one on marriage was for me. Everything I knew about women came from one-night stands and casual dating relationships inundated with my own selfishness and sexual sin. I was determined to change, so I suspected that the marriage class would be the perfect place to learn how men and women were meant to relate.

I didn't date during that year under Joel's teaching, hoping this would also help me reset my approach to women. I might have been the only man in history to attend a married-couples' class for most of a year without even having a single date! But just before the nine-month mark, I prayed this simple prayer: "Lord, I've been in this class for months and learned a lot about the characteristics of godly women, but I'm not sure I've ever seen these qualities in real life. I've never really known any Christian girls. Please show me a woman who embodies these traits."

I wasn't asking for a date, girlfriend, or spouse. I just wanted to see these qualities in real life so that I might understand them better.

God gave me far more than that: one week later He introduced me to Brenda! She was absolutely fascinating to me. I could see in her all the glorious characteristics I'd been learning about during those nine months, and the more I got to know Brenda, the more desperately I desired to be worthy of her and live up to God's standards as a man. It wasn't long until we fell in love and wanted to marry.

Out of our commitment to Christ, Brenda and I decided to stay pure before marriage. She was a virgin, and I wished I was. We did kiss, however, and whoa! Our smooching was wonderful! It was my first experience of something that I'll call the paradox of obedience: the physically gratifying payoff that comes from obedience to God's sexual standards.

In explanation, consider this thought: In a song made popular by Eric Carmen during my senior year in college, the singer mourned about trying to remember how it used to feel when a kiss was something special. The lyrics from the song resonated sadly with me because, at that point in my life, a kiss meant nothing to me. It was a joyless prerequisite on the path to intercourse. But now with Brenda, having cut the physical things way back to obey God's standards, a simple kiss with her was thrilling again. To an old sex hog like me, this was a totally unexpected and pleasant surprise. I was learning how good His ways were for me.

As God continued to work in my life, Brenda and I married, honeymooned in Colorado, and then settled into a new apartment building. Was this heaven? I surely thought so.

I threw myself into my sales career and leadership roles at church. Then I became a dad. I relished it all, and my image as a Christian shined brighter and brighter. By most standards, I was doing great. Just one little problem: by *God's* standard of sexual purity, I wasn't close to living out His vision for marriage.

Sure, while once I was engaged to two women at the same time, now I was happily married to one woman. And while before I was drowning in pornography, now I hadn't purchased a pornographic magazine since before my wedding day. Given my track record, this was remarkable. But did these changes make me sexually pure? Hardly. As God's child, I was to have no hint of sexual immorality in my life. Although I'd certainly taken steps toward purity, I was learning that God's standards were higher than I'd ever imagined and that my Father had higher hopes for me than I had dreamed.

Stopping Short

It soon became clear that I'd stopped far too short of holiness. There were the Sunday-morning ad inserts, of course, and the double entendres and heat-seeking eyes. There were the movies and the masturbation while away on road trips. My mind daydreamed and fantasized over former girlfriends and dwelled too long on the pretty faces and shapes of the women at work. These were more than a hint of sexual immorality. I was paying heavy prices for these fantasies, and the bills were piling up. My intimacy with God was fading.

People around me disagreed with my assessment, saying, "Oh, come on, that can't be the reason you feel distant from God! Those are just little things you're doing, just part of being a guy. Nobody can control their eyes and mind! God loves you. It must be something else." But I knew differently.

As I mentioned earlier, I'd already found it difficult to connect with the Lord in worship, but now I couldn't even seem to look Him in the eye in prayer. After all, I kept making these tearful promises to Him that I'd clean up my act, but I kept breaking those vows again and again. I was a hypocrite and a liar. *How could He possibly care to hear from me even one more time in prayer?* I wondered. At the time, I couldn't believe that He did.

My prayer life grew feeble. Once, our son Jasen became very sick and was rushed to the emergency room. Did I rush into prayer? No, I could only rush others to pray. "Have you called our pastor to pray?" I asked Brenda. "Have you called Ron and Red?" I had no faith in my own prayers because of my sin.

At church I was an empty suit. I went to church desperately needing ministry and forgiveness and *never* arrived ready to minister to others. After all, I'd been "preparing" for church by lusting and masturbating over lingerie ads. My prayers were no more effective in God's house than anywhere else.

As a full-commission salesperson, if I lost a number of deals in a row to the competition, I could never be sure if those setbacks weren't somehow caused by my sin. I had no peace.

I was personally paying a heavy spiritual price for my sin.

My marriage was suffering as well. Brenda had come from four generations of passionate lovers of God, and I believed that if she ever found out about these things that I was doing in secret, she'd leave me. Because of my sin, I couldn't commit 100 percent to Brenda, out of fear that if she dumped me, I'd be 100 percent destroyed emotionally. That cost Brenda in closeness.

But that's not all. Sometimes at dawn, when I was in the very act of lusting over those lingerie ads, I'd hear Brenda dashing down the stairs from the master bedroom to find me in the family room. She'd still be gasping in terror and in tears after experiencing yet another frightening nightmare in which she was being chased by Satan. "Fred, where were you?" she'd wail. "I was running down long, dark hallways, and Satan was chasing me and getting closer and closer! I opened every door, looking for you to defend me. Where were you?" Then she'd drop into my chest, sobbing hysterically in panic and dread.

How do you think I felt in those moments? Try *horrible*! I knew my immorality was compromising my spiritual protection over Brenda, allowing the Enemy to pick on her in her dreams. (In case you're wondering, Brenda never had another dream like that once I'd gained my victory over sexual sin.)

During those days, my pastor was preaching a series about generational sin—patterns of sin passed from father to son (see Exodus 34:7). Sitting in my pew, I recalled that my grandfather had run off from his wife in the middle of the Great Depression, leaving her with six kids. My own father left our family to pursue multiple sexual affairs and a pornographic, *Playboy*-inspired lifestyle. That same pattern had been passed on to me, proven by my deep dive into the same foul pornographic pools and my chase after multiple girlfriends.

And now my cherubic firstborn son, Jasen, was toddling over to me endlessly with his happy, drippy grins and shining eyes that gushed, *Daddy, I want to grow up to be just like you!*

Seeing Jasen, I would scream silently, *No, son! Don't grow up to be like me! I can't free myself from this sexual prison. Don't imitate me!* Though saved, I still didn't have this purity issue settled in my life, and I was petrified by the thought of passing this pattern on to my kids.

Perhaps no one else saw it, but I could no longer miss the connection between my sexual immorality and my distance from God. Since I'd already cut out the porn and had no desire for intimacy with anyone but my wife, I looked pretty pure on the outside to others. But to God, I'd merely stopped short at a false finish line in mushy middle ground, resting somewhere between paganism and obedience to God's standard.

Desperation

The Lord desired more for me. He had freed me through salvation, and while I was eternally grateful for that, I was realizing that I had never really taken that good, long bath I needed to get fully clean. In short, I'd stopped moving toward Him, and my sanctification had stalled.

I had expected the journey of purity to be easier than this. I'd figured I could easily get rid of all the sexual junk in my life. But I couldn't. Every week I said I wouldn't look at those ad inserts, but every Sunday morning, the striking photos compelled me to lust. Every week I'd vow to avoid watching R-rated "sexy" movies when I traveled on business, but every week I'd fail, sweating out tough battles of temptation and always losing. Every time I gazed at some glistening jogger bouncing by, I'd promise to never do it again. But I always did.

What I'd done was simply trade the pornography of *Playboy* and *Gallery* for the pornography of ad inserts and other magazine ads. I wasn't considering physical extramarital affairs, but I was certainly having *mental* affairs and daydreams—affairs of the eyes and heart.

In short, while the pornography was gone, the sin remained. I'd never really escaped the sexual slavery. I'd never truly rejected my visual feasting upon women. I'd merely changed where I went for a meal.

A couple of months slipped by, then a couple of years. The distance from God grew wider, the bills stacked higher, and my impurity still ruled me. My faith waned further with each failure. Each desperate loss led to deeper desolation. While I could always say, "No more," I could never mean it.

Something was gripping me—something relentless, something mean.

Still, against all odds, I eventually found total freedom, just like Steve Arterburn. Since then, both Steve and I have had the chance to talk to countless men hopelessly ensnared in their own sensual pigsties, just as desperate to be free. Now that we've shared our stories, we're going to share a few of theirs in the next chapter, hoping you'll relate to not just their struggles but also their victories over sin and their paths to freedom.

3

Addiction? Or Something Else?

Before you experience victory over sexual sin, you're hurting and confused. *Why can't I win this battle?* you snarl in frustration. As the fight wears on and the losses pile higher, you may begin to doubt everything about yourself, perhaps even your salvation. At best, you think that you're deeply flawed; at worst, an evil person. You probably feel very alone, since men rarely speak openly about these things.

But you're not alone. Countless men have fallen into their own sexual pits, as you are about to see.

From Fred: Are You Noticing?

These pitfalls happen easily since there is so much sexual immorality in our society. We get desensitized to it and sometimes don't recognize it for what it is.

One day a fellow named Mike was telling me about renting the video *Forrest Gump*. "Boy, it was great!" he exclaimed. "Tom Hanks was brilliant, which is why he won the Oscar for Best Actor. I laughed and cried all the way through it. I know Brenda and you rent good movies for your kids. You should get this one. It was really clean and wholesome."

"Oh, I can't watch *Forrest Gump* with my kids. In fact, I can't even watch that myself, Mike," I responded.

Taken aback, Mike asked, "Why? It was a great movie!"

"Well, do you remember that scene at the beginning where Sally Field has sex with the principal to get her son into the 'right' school?"

"Uh . . ."

"And how about the bare breasts at the New Year's party? The nude on-stage guitar performance? And in the end, when Forrest finally 'got the girl' in the sex scene and she conceived a child out of wedlock? Sure, in the movie, everything worked out nicely for Forrest anyway. But that normally isn't how life goes in those situations, so I don't want to teach that to my kids. I don't want them to hear all that grunting or see the nudity, either."

Mike slumped into a chair. "I guess I've been watching movies for so long that I didn't even notice those things."

How about you? Are you noticing such things, or have you been desensitized too? Think about it. Suppose you drop your kids at Grandma's for the weekend and decide to access your Netflix account and watch *Forrest Gump* with your wife. You pop some corn, put your arm around her, and click Play. After much laughter and tears, you both agree that *Forrest Gump* was a great movie.

But you got more than entertainment, didn't you? You remember the grunting and panting between Sally Field and the principal and how when Sally Field next appeared on screen, you briefly looked her up and down and wondered what it might be like to have her under the sheets. You had your arm around your wife while you were thinking it. Then later, after you retired to bed for a "bit of sport," you replaced your wife's face and body with Sally Field's, and you wondered why she couldn't make you grunt and pant like the principal.

"Come on!" you reply. "This stuff happens all the time." Could be, but listen to these troubling words from Jesus: "I tell you that anyone who looks at a woman lustfully has already committed adultery with her in his heart" (Matthew 5:28).

In light of this scripture, piddling things like objecting to *Forrest Gump* may not be minor, legalistic meddling. Such subtle influences, added to hundreds of others over time, provide us with more than a hint of sexual immorality. Soon the effect isn't so subtle and isn't as fun.

Struggles All Around

Let us share some other stories with you.

Thad is recovering from drug dependency at a local Christian ministry. "I've been trying hard to get my life in order," he said. "At the drug center, I've learned more about myself and my addiction to drugs. I expected that, since that's why I went there. But I've discovered a second, unexpected thing: I have a problem with lust and impurity.

"I want to be free, but I'm becoming frustrated and angry with the church. The Bible says that women should dress modestly, but they don't. Some women on the worship team wear the latest tight, short skirts. I look at them worshipping God, but what I see are curves and legs. I get frustrated that how women dress can make purity harder for me even though I'm right there in church where I should be."

Howard, a Sunday school teacher, described a life-twisting event in junior high: "I was walking home with a classmate named Billy. I didn't really like Billy that much, but I felt sorry for him. He didn't have many friends, and he was trying so hard to make some. On our way to buy a drink at a convenience store, he told me about something called masturbation. I'd never heard that word, so he explained what it was. He said all the guys had been experimenting with it.

"I couldn't get what he told me out of my mind, so that night I tried it. Since then, more than fifteen years ago, I haven't gone more than a week without masturbating!

"I always thought marriage would take the desire away, but it isn't any better and I'm so ashamed. Not so much by the act itself, but by the things I think about and the movies I watch while doing it. I know it's adulterous."

Another guy, named Joe, told us he loves women's beach volleyball. "At night, I've had shockingly vivid dreams of these women," he confided. "Some have been so exhilarating and so real that I wake up the next morning certain that I've been in bed with them. It's so real that I feel guilt, wondering where my wife is—I'm sure she has left me over this affair—and how I could've done such a thing. Finally, as the cobwebs clear, it slowly dawns on me that it was just a dream. But even then, I feel uneasy. You want to know why? Because while I know it was just a dream, I'm not at all certain it wasn't some form of adultery."

Wally, a businessman and frequent traveler, told us he absolutely dreads hotels. "I always eat a long, leisurely dinner," he says, "stalling before returning to my room, because I know what's coming. Before too long, I have the TV remote in my hand. I tell myself it'll be for only a minute, but I know I'm lying. I know what I really want. I'm hoping to catch a little sex scene or two as I search the channels. I tell myself that I'll watch for only a while or that I'll stop before I get carried away. Then my motor gets going and I lust for more, sometimes even turning to the X-rated channel.

"The RPMs are going so high that I have to do something or it feels like my engine will blow. So I masturbate. On a few occasions I fight it, but if I do, later on when I turn the lights out, I'm flooded with lustful thoughts and desires. I stare wide eyed at the ceiling. I see nothing, but I literally feel the bombardment, the throbbing desire. I have no way to get to sleep, and it's killing me. So I say, 'Okay, if I masturbate, I'll have peace and I can finally get to sleep.' So I do, and guess what? The guilt is so strong that I still can't get to sleep. I wake up totally exhausted in the morning.

"What's wrong with me? Do other men have this problem? I'm afraid to ask, really. What if this isn't how everyone else is? What would that say about me? Worse, what if this is how everyone else is? What would that say about the guys at my church?"

John wakes up early to watch certain exercise videos on YouTube, though he doesn't care much about fitness. "The truth is," he began, "I feel absolutely compelled to watch, to catch the close-ups of the buttocks, the breasts, and especially the inner thighs, and I lust and lust and lust. I sometimes wonder if the producers doing those close-ups are just trying to hook men into watching their shows.

"Every day I tell myself that this will be the last time. But by next morning, I'm right there at the computer again."

These men are not weirdos. They are your next-door neighbors, your fellow workers, even your in-laws. They are you. They are small-group leaders, ushers, and deacons. Even pastors aren't immune. One young pastor tearfully detailed to us his ministry and his desire to serve God, expressing in a deeply moving way his devotion to his call. But his tears turned to wrenching sobs as he spoke of his bondage to pornography and how it hinders his ministry. His spirit is willing, but his flesh is weak.

Spinning in the Cycles

What about you? Maybe it's true that when you and a woman reach a door simultaneously, you wait to let her go first, but not out of honor. You want to follow her up the stairs and look her over. Maybe you've driven your rental car to the parking lot of a local gym between appointments, watching scantily clad women bouncing in and out, fantasizing and lusting—even masturbating—in the car. Maybe you can't stay away from Sixth Avenue, where the prostitutes ply their trade. Not that you'd ever hire one. Or maybe you don't want to sneak a look at porn sites on your smartphone, but when sitting alone in your cubicle, you just can't help yourself.

You're still teaching a children's Sunday school class, still playing guitar for a worship team, still going to the men's group, still supporting your family. You've been faithful to your wife—well, at least you haven't had an actual physical affair. You're getting ahead, living in a nice home with nice cars and nice clothes and a nice future. *People look to me as an example,* you reason. *I'm okay.*

Yet privately, your conscience dims until you can't quite tell what's right or wrong anymore, watching the latest Hollywood releases without even noticing the sexuality. You're choking in the sexual prison you've made, wondering where the promises of God have gone. You spin in the same sinful cycles year after year.

And nagging you is the worship. The prayer times. The distance. Always the distance from God. Meanwhile, your sexual sin remains so consistent that you can set your watch by it.

Rick, for instance, walks down the hall at break time just to glance through the glass doors of another office where a sexy young administrative assistant answers phones and directs clients. "Every morning at nine thirty, I wave at her and she smiles back," he says wistfully. "She's beautiful, and her clothes—let's just say they really accentuate her best features. I don't know her name, but I'm actually disappointed when she's absent from work."

Similarly, Sid races home by 4 p.m. every summer day. That's when his neighbor

Angela sunbathes right outside his window. "At four o'clock, she lies out in a bikini, and she doesn't know I can see her. I can gaze to my heart's content. She's so sexy I can hardly stand it, and I masturbate every day when I watch her."

And what of today, twenty years after *Every Man's Battle* was first released? Please recall what we wrote in the introduction: "Pornographers have grown more vile and more depraved in the last twenty years, [which means the material they produce] is vastly more vicious and twisted, inflicting a dramatic deterioration in a guy's ability to even get an erection and perform sexually in the master bedroom."

Because of these changes, the stories we're hearing these days are even grislier than those we mentioned earlier. Jacob, a Christian twentysomething, told me that after watching porn videos for a couple of years, he met a beautiful woman at work. "She was pretty provocative. I knew she was open to anything, so I took her out of town on a three-day weekend to a nice resort. The room came with a hot tub on the balcony and a giant round bed—the works. I did everything to her I'd ever seen in my porn videos, and she did the same to me. She told me that I was 'way great,' but you know something? When the long weekend was over, it really hit me: I hadn't felt a thing."

Jacob sought to find the intensity he'd felt watching his sexy videos, but he couldn't conjure up the same passion with a real woman anymore, even in a glorious resort hotel room, because she couldn't take him where his hands and fantasies had taken him with porn. In short, porn and masturbation had crept in and taken over his sexual makeup, eventually frying his natural inclinations to a crisp. We see it happening to men at an accelerated pace.

Sure, porn has always been able to push you into bizarre, irresponsible thought patterns about sex with real women. But that now seems quaint when compared to the effects of today's escalated pornographic themes, which warp and pull at your sexual horizons until you can enjoy pornography in all sorts of different configurations, sometimes involving a couple of men, sometimes a woman with a German shepherd, perhaps with a woman and several guys, or even with a frantic, resistant girl being ravished and forcefully subdued before your eyes. You can find every sort of image you could ever imagine in these videos and even more that you would never have imagined. In fact, it's become irrefutably clear that the internet doesn't just *re-*

veal your sexual tastes but also *creates* them, well outside your consciousness, as you surf from site to site. If anything loses its appeal, you simply bounce up to the next level, which is often more intense and, usually, more violent.

Before long, you're just one more statistic in a brand-new epidemic among twenty- and thirtysomethings called porn-induced erectile dysfunction (PIED). No, you don't have low testosterone, and no, you haven't broken your penis by overusing it for hours at a time while online. Your penis still works fine, as long as you're in front of a computer.

What you've actually "broken" is another sex organ—your brain, which is widely considered the largest sexual organ in a man's body. To be perfectly accurate, of course, you haven't broken it but rewired it. Extensive porn use induces long-term neuroplastic change in the brain that literally alters how sexual pleasure is routed and processed there. That is why you struggle to *get* an erection with your wife, even though she's got what it takes and is forever the love of your life. That's why you struggle to *keep* an erection, even when you've forced her to perform like a porn star for you.

We intend to demystify this entire topic for you. By the time you turn the last page in this book, you will know exactly how the brain gets rewired by your sin, and you'll know exactly how to reverse the effects. Whether you are married or single, you can apply these principles and get back on purity's track.

Let's get started by addressing the most basic question on this battlefield.

The Big Question

Are these men sex addicts? The compelling sexual cravings are certainly strong evidence. Still, let's take a quick historical look at the study of sexual addiction in men to get a better idea of what addiction means for our purposes in this book.

When we published *Every Man's Battle* in 1999, sexual addiction was a fairly new area of human biological science. In fact, the earliest book on the topic had only been released in 1983, *Out of the Shadows* by Patrick Carnes. As I finished writing and editing my *own* manuscript, I picked up a copy of that book at the suggestion of my publisher.

During those early days, researchers and counselors were simply attempting to get their arms around the range of behaviors involved, and Carnes had helpfully devised a grid of behavioral levels to help arrive at a clinical definition of sexual addiction.

As a matter of fact, Steve and I used his clinical definition as a starting point in the original version of *Every Man's Battle,* and we'll use it again now to mark out the place where most men live when it comes to their compelling sexual cravings.

From Fred: A Thunderbolt

I vividly remember the merciless internal struggles between the consequences of my sin and the pleasures of my sin. Yes, I hated my sin and cursed it at my core, as most Christian men do. Still, it seemed that no matter how painfully that sin ripped across my heart and soul, it could never quite trump the pleasure of the sin, so I couldn't—or wouldn't—stop. My sexual desires owned me lock, stock, and barrel. It's the same with the men whose stories I've just shared. Maybe you're owned too.

But did I qualify as an addict? Many guys ask a similar question.

The answer? Well, that's complicated. Let me explain. When I first read Carnes's description of a four-step addiction cycle—preoccupation, ritualization, compulsive sexual behavior, then despair—I knew I'd lived that pattern.[*] From that perspective, I was certain that what I'd experienced was addiction.

But a thunderbolt hit me when this same writer went on to state a clinical definition of sexual addiction by using his three levels of addictive behavior[†] (keep in mind that this isn't a Christian book):

Level 1: "Behaviors that are regarded as normal, acceptable, or tolerable. Examples include masturbation, pornography, and prostitution."

Level 2: "Behaviors which are clearly victimizing and for which legal sanctions are enforced. These are generally seen as nuisance offenses, such as exhibitionism or voyeurism."

---

[*] Patrick J. Carnes, PhD, *Out of the Shadows: Understanding Sexual Addiction*, 3rd ed. (Center City, MN: Hazelden, 2001) 19–20.

[†] Carnes, *Out of the Shadows*, 37.

Level 3: "Behaviors [that] have grave consequences for the victims and legal consequences for the addicts; examples are incest, child molestation, or rape."

Did you read that list closely? I sure did, and I noticed that the examples of level 1 include not just masturbation, which most men practice at times (to me, masturbation seemed out of place here at level 1, unless you're talking compulsive masturbation, done many times a day), but also homosexuality and prostitution.

It struck me that most men grappling with bad sexual habits never actually reach this first level of addiction. Defining sexual addiction this way may make perfect sense from a clinical point of view in the counseling arena, but my own experience on the battlefield convinced me that these levels didn't apply to the men I knew at church. Sure, viewing pornography and masturbating were rampant among my Christian brothers, but not to a compulsive degree. And homosexuality? Prostitution? In some cases, sure, but not with the vast majority.

So, judging by Carnes's clinical definition of sexual addiction, maybe I wasn't an addict after all. Clearly, you can live out the preoccupation, ritualization, compulsive sexual behavior, and despair of the addiction cycle—like I'd done—without ever moving up to one of these three levels of addictive behavior.

But if I wasn't an addict and the other guys I've mentioned in this chapter weren't addicts, what *were* we?

From Steve: Fractional Addiction

To help answer that question, let's think again about those three levels of addiction as described above. From our Christian perspective, let's insert another level at the bottom of the addiction scale. If we categorized being totally pure and holy as the zero level, most Christian men we know would fall somewhere between level 0 and level 1.

If you're one of the many men living at this level, it probably isn't at all helpful to label you as an addict in the clinical sense or imply that victory will take years of therapy, because it won't. Instead, victory can be measured in weeks and months, as we'll describe later.

Not all "addictive" behaviors are rooted in some deep, dark, shadowy mental maze of crushing emotional pain and past abuse, as they often are with men in levels 1, 2, and 3. Rather, your behaviors may be based on pleasure highs. Obviously, because of the way we've been created, men receive a chemical high from sexually charged images.

The hormone epinephrine is part of this pleasure chemistry. It's secreted into the bloodstream and locks into the memory whatever sensual stimulus you're viewing at the time of the emotional excitement. In fact, epinephrine can be released merely by using your *mind's* eye. I've counseled men who became emotionally and sexually stimulated just from entertaining thoughts of sexual activity. For instance, a guy dead set on perusing his favorite porn sites is sexually stimulated long before he taps on a certain app to conduct a search. His stimulation begins in his thought process (the mind's eye), which triggers his nervous system, which secretes epinephrine into the bloodstream, which leads him to pick up his smartphone.

Over the past twenty years, brain science has further detailed much of the brain chemistry involved in these addictive patterns that bind us, which is a key reason why we are updating *Every Man's Battle.* We'll share a lot more about that in chapter 6. For right now, it is enough to understand that pleasure chemicals lie at the root of our compulsive sexual behavior.

From my counseling experience, I believe a lot of those men living at the upper levels have psychological problems that will take years to work through. Even then, a life of sexual integrity could start now. But the majority of men don't live there. Again, our contention is that the vast majority of men stuck in sexual sin are living between level 0 and level 1.

Fred and I call this a fractional addiction, since it represents living at a level that's a fraction between zero and one. When we're fractionally addicted, we surely experience powerful and seemingly irresistible addictive drawings, but we aren't generally compelled to act to salve some pain, at least not in the same intensity as the men at those higher levels of addiction. Instead, we're more compelled by the chemical high and the sexual gratification it brings.

I lived in this area of fractional addiction during my first decade of marriage, as well as earlier in my adolescence and college years. My interest in the female body had been formed when I was around five years old and was visiting my grandfather's machine shop in Ranger, Texas. I loved walking into that old shop filled with lathes and presses, where Grandpa made tools to retrieve broken oil-well pipes. His office wall was adorned with nude pinups, and I stared at those voluptuous naked women in awe.

As I grew older, I saw women more as objects than as people who had feelings. Pornography became for me an enticement to forbidden love. Many young women I dated in high school and college were sexually pure and stayed sexually pure while we dated, but I was always manipulating and conniving, going for what was forbidden.

I later tasted the forbidden fruit when I entered the promiscuous period of my life. When I did have premarital sex, it gave me a sense of connection, as if these young women accepted me fully. They were there for my validation as a man, and sadly I used them just as my grandfather had used those pictures on the wall of his shop.

What I needed to do was train my eyes and mind to behave, just as Fred did. I needed to align my eyes and mind with Scripture and avoid every hint of sexual immorality. But before we get into an action plan for realigning our eyes and minds, we need to talk further about the roots of this sexual bondage.

Why We Live There

While the concept of fractional addiction has been helpful in explaining where most of us Christian men live, it doesn't explain why we live there and in such vast numbers. While it is notoriously difficult, for a number of reasons, to conduct research on porn, the Barna Group found that even 57 percent of pastors and 64 percent of youth pastors admit to struggling with pornography from time to time.[*]

On the surface, this doesn't make sense. After all, as Christians we've all given our lives to God and have committed to live according to His ways. His standard of sexual purity is part of His ways. Why, then, do nearly all of us live in this state of fractional addiction, when most of us don't want to live there and few of us made a conscious decision to go there in the first place?

---

[*] David Kinnaman, *The Porn Phenomenon*, Barna, February 5, 2016, www.barna.com/the-porn-phenomenon.

Hmmm. Stop right there for a moment and analyze what was just said. We didn't *want* to go there and did not *choose* to go there, yet nearly *all* of us end up there.

That is telling, isn't it? And it can mean only one thing. There must be something *inside* our makeup as men that makes us particularly susceptible to sexual addiction, and there must be something *outside* us in our culture that makes this whole slippery slope so slick.

That something inside you is your makeup as a male, including the ability of the male eye to deliver sexually gratifying pleasure chemicals to the brain when it locks on to the sensual objects in its vicinity. That something outside is a culture that's locked in on making sure that everything around you is crammed full of sensuality to flood your pleasure centers, from the bouncy babe at the beach in her thong bikini to the steamy hot flicks at the Cinépolis movie theaters to the voluptuous, duck-lipped classmate sexting topless selfies straight to your smartphone.

The question of whether or not you officially qualify as an addict is much less important than understanding that these drives are chemically charged and therefore seem impossible to resist. If we are ever going to get free, we must first explore our makeup as men and why our sensual culture is so compelling to us in spite of our love for Christ. Only then will we be able to defend ourselves from sexual addiction, so let's study our male makeup together in the next section.

One final note: Addiction or no addiction, the concepts and principles presented here work for both. If you are wondering if it is sin or addiction, the answer is "yes"! All have sinned, and every addict has sin in many areas of life. I've never met an addict without sin. And as for sinners, I've never met one who isn't addicted to his or her favorite sin.

Part II

How We Got Here

4

Mixing Standards

For most of us men, becoming ensnared by sexual sin happens easily and naturally, like slipping off an icy log. Why is that? It's because we are easy marks. After all, we have two natural elements in our physical makeup as men that set us up to fall effortlessly into sexual sin if we're not taught early how to make a stand.

Let's stop right there. It can be too easy to breeze by the early paragraphs of a new chapter without genuine focus, so let's slow down a moment to ponder what that last paragraph really says, which is this: *Our created, physical makeup as men sets us up to fall into sexual sin without conscious effort when we live in a sensual, sex-drenched culture like this one.*

You've *got* to realize this if you expect to defend yourself effectively, and you must grasp how these two natural elements work together to make you easy pickings in the battle. Let's flag these elements right now.

First of all, as guys we more naturally run to the *world* for our values and beliefs instead of to the *Word*. This is a tendency that's rooted in our male brain structure and instinctively dominates our interactions with the guys around us.

Our second natural vulnerability to sexual sin rests in how our eyes and brains process sexual pleasure. These two aspects of our male makeup help explain the high percentage of Christian men trapped by sexual sin in spite of their love for God.

We can think back upon our early lives as guys to see how easily this happens. Most of us slip into sexual sin during our teen years before we even know what's going on. Because we're set up to fall by nature, we don't need to make a grand, conscious decision to rebel against God's standards—it just happens rather easily, like when we wander into our grandfather's office with the voluptuous nudes on the wall or we stumble across our dad's *Playboy* magazine under his bed or a friend describes something called masturbation and we innocently try it out of curiosity. In this culture, there are a multitude of ways to get tripped up, made much easier because of internet porn and smartphones.

Interestingly, because many of us slipped into sexual sin without making a deliberate choice, we were more puzzled by it than concerned. We didn't yet realize exactly what we'd tumbled into or that we had a battle on our hands. Since we lacked understanding of the addictive nature of sexual sin, we assumed our escape from it would be as effortless as that first step into the trap.

From Fred: Misplaced Confidence

So, most guys expect to grow out of sexual temptation as naturally as they grew into it—like outgrowing acne. Perhaps you waited with each birthday for your sexual impurity to clear up, like I did. But that never happened.

Later, perhaps you assumed that marriage would naturally free you, without a fight. But—as for many of us—that didn't happen either.

When Mark signed up for my premarriage class, he told me, "The whole problem of impurity has been a mess. I've been hooked for years, and I'm counting on marriage to free me. I'll be able to have sex whenever I want it. Then Satan won't be able to tempt me at all!"

When Mark and I got together a few years later, I wasn't surprised to hear that marriage hadn't fixed the problem. "You know, Fred, my wife doesn't desire sex as often as I do," he said.

Oh, really?

"I don't want to seem like a sex addict or anything, but I probably have as many unmet desires now as I did before marriage. On top of all that, some areas of sexual exploration seem embarrassing or immodest to her. Sometimes she even calls them kinky. I think she's rather prudish, so what should I say to her?"

In my experience, not much!

Marriage: No Sexual Nirvana

That marriage doesn't eliminate sexual impurity comes as no surprise to married men, although it does for teens and young singles. Bowen, a youth pastor in Minnesota, said that when he challenges young men to be sexually pure, their response is, "That's easy for you to say, Pastor. You're married. You can have sex anytime you want!" Young singles believe that marriage creates a state of sexual nirvana. If only it were so.

But why isn't it so?

The answer is pretty easy in retrospect. First of all, sex has different meanings to men and women. Men primarily receive intimacy just before and during intercourse. Women gain intimacy through touching, sharing, hugging, and communication. Is it any wonder that the frequency of sex is less important to women than to men, as Mark woefully discovered? Because of the differences between men and women, forming a satisfying sex life in marriage is hardly a slam dunk; it's more like making a half-court shot.

Second, life throws hard curves. Lance married his sweetheart, only to find that she had a structural problem that made intercourse very painful. It took surgery and months of rehabilitation to correct it. For Jayden, his wife once became so ill that they couldn't have intercourse for eight months. Did these circumstances free Lance and Jayden to say, *God, I'll just keep using porn and masturbation until You heal my wife?* We don't think so.

Third, your wife may suddenly become much different from the woman you courted. Larry, a strapping, handsome young pastor in Washington, DC, has a great Christian heritage. His father was a wonderful pastor, and Larry was thrilled when God also called him into the ministry. When Larry met Linda, a striking blond bombshell, they appeared meant for each other, a regular Ken-and-Barbie set.

After their wedding day, however, Larry found Linda to be far more interested in her career than in fulfilling him sexually. Not only was she disinterested in sex, but she often used it as a manipulative weapon to get her way. Consequently, Larry didn't have sex very often. Twice a month was a bonanza, and once every two months was the norm.

What's Larry supposed to say to God? *Lord, Linda is being ungodly! Change her, and then I'll stop masturbating!* Hardly. Marriage didn't satisfy Larry's sexual needs, but God still expects purity (just as God would expect Linda to change, as her actions are *also* way off biblical course and must be called sin). Your purity must not depend upon your mate's health or sexual desire. God holds *you* responsible, and if you don't gain control of your sexuality before your wedding day, you can expect the same old bondage to wrap you up after the honeymoon. If you're single and watching sensual R-rated movies regularly, wedded bliss won't erase this habit. If your eyes lock on passing babes, they'll still roam after you say "I do." You're masturbating now? Putting that ring on your finger won't keep your hands off yourself.

What's Going On Here?

So, you haven't naturally grown out of your sexual sin, and marriage hasn't solved your problem either. But perhaps you're still clinging to one last hope that, given enough time, marriage may yet free you naturally, without a battle.

Andy told us, "I once read that a man's sex drive drops in his thirties and forties, while a woman's sex drive reaches its peak during that time. For a while, I thought that Jill and I would meet in some blissful middle ground. It didn't happen."

Look, it's time you dump the false hopes and accept the truth. Your male makeup made those first, subconscious steps down the slippery slope easy and effortless, but because of that same male makeup, a return to the summit will never happen without a fight. If you're tired of sexual impurity and the mediocre, distant relationship with God that results from it, quit waiting on marriage or some hormone drop to save the day.

If you want to change, you'll have to fight for it. Freedom is never free. Purity will cost you something. You'll need to man up, find your vulnerabilities, and then defend against them with all your heart. Expect a battle. That's the road back to the summit.

God's Standard from the Bible

To fight your way back, you must start by recognizing that you're impure because, somewhere along life's way, you've diluted God's standard of sexual purity with your own, by choice or by chance. We said earlier that God's standard is that we avoid every hint of sexual immorality in our lives. Had you followed this standard from boyhood, you'd have never seen sexual bondage, in spite of your male makeup.

It's clear, then, if you're to win this war, you must reverse course and go God's way. You must *stop* mixing God's standard of sexual purity with your own ideas, and you must *start* avoiding every hint of sexual impurity in your life.

And since that is the path to victory, it's vital we take a moment to outline God's standards more completely so that you know exactly where you're aiming, because today many men have no clue about God's standard for sexual purity or even what it looks like to avoid every hint of sexual immorality.

The following is a selection of verses in the New Testament that teach of God's concern for our sexual purity. Italics show key words indicating what we're to avoid in the sexual realm.

I [Jesus] tell you that anyone who *looks at a woman lustfully* has already committed adultery with her in his heart. (Matthew 5:28)

It is from within, out of a person's heart, that evil thoughts come—*sexual immorality,* theft, murder, *adultery,* greed, malice, deceit, *lewdness,* envy, slander, arrogance and folly. All these evils come from inside and defile a person. (Mark 7:21–23)

You are to abstain from . . . *sexual immorality.* (Acts 15:29)

Let us put aside the deeds of darkness and put on the armor of light. Let us behave decently, as in the daytime, not in *carousing* and drunkenness, not in *sexual immorality* and *debauchery,* not in dissension and jealousy. (Romans 13:12–13)

I am writing to you that you must not associate with anyone who claims to be a brother or sister but is *sexually immoral* or greedy, an idolater or a slanderer, a drunkard or a swindler. Do not even eat with such people. (1 Corinthians 5:11)

The body . . . is not meant for *sexual immorality* but for the Lord. (1 Corinthians 6:13)

Flee from *sexual immorality.* (1 Corinthians 6:18)

I am afraid that when I come again . . . I will be grieved over many who have sinned earlier and have not repented of the *impurity, sexual sin* and *debauchery* in which they have indulged. (2 Corinthians 12:21)

Walk by the Spirit, and you will not gratify the desires of the flesh. . . . The acts of the flesh are obvious: sexual immorality, impurity and debauchery. (Galatians 5:16, 19)

Among you there must not be even a hint of *sexual immorality,* or of any kind of *impurity,* or of greed, because these are improper for God's holy people. Nor should there be *obscenity,* foolish talk or coarse joking, which are out of place. (Ephesians 5:3–4)

Put to death . . . whatever belongs to your earthly nature: *sexual immorality, impurity, lust, evil desires* and greed, which is idolatry. Because of these, the wrath of God is coming. (Colossians 3:5–6)

It is God's will that you should be sanctified: that you should avoid *sexual immorality;* that each of you should learn to control your own body in a way that is holy and honorable, not in *passionate lust* like the pagans, who do not know God. . . . For God did not call us to be *impure,* but to live a holy life. (1 Thessalonians 4:3–5, 7)

See that no one is *sexually immoral.* (Hebrews 12:16)

Marriage should be honored by all, and the marriage bed kept pure, for God will judge the *adulterer* and all the *sexually immoral.* (Hebrews 13:4)

You have spent enough time in the past doing what pagans choose to do—
living in *debauchery, lust,* drunkenness, *orgies,* carousing and detestable
idolatry. (1 Peter 4:3)

Sodom and Gomorrah and the surrounding towns gave themselves up to
sexual immorality and perversion. They serve as an example of those who suf-
fer the punishment of eternal fire. (Jude 7)

I [Jesus] have a few things against you: There are some among you who hold
to the teaching of Balaam, who taught Balak to entice the Israelites to sin so
that they . . . committed *sexual immorality.* (Revelation 2:14)

I [Jesus] have this against you: You tolerate that woman Jezebel, who calls
herself a prophet. By her teaching she misleads my servants into *sexual immorality.* (Revelation 2:20)

The cowardly, the unbelieving, the vile, the murderers, the *sexually immoral,*
those who practice magic arts, the idolaters and all liars—they will be con-
signed to the fiery lake of burning sulfur. This is the second death. (Revelation 21:8)

Isn't that amazing? More than half the books in the New Testament are represented here, so while we can all agree that some topics in Scripture are confusing, our
call to sexual integrity isn't one of them.

Drawing from these passages, let's summarize God's standard for sexual purity:

- Sexual immorality begins with the lustful attitudes of our sinful nature. It is rooted in the darkness within us. Therefore, sexual immorality, like other sins that enslave, will incur God's wrath.
- Our bodies were not meant for sexual immorality but for the Lord,
  who has both created us and called us to live in sexual purity. His
  will is that every Christian be sexually pure—in his thoughts and
  his words, as well as in his actions.

- Therefore, it is holy and honorable to completely avoid sexual immorality—to repent of it, to flee from it, and to put it to death in our lives as we live by the Spirit. We've spent enough time living in passionate lust like pagans. It's time to change.
- We shouldn't be in close association with another Christian who persists in sexual immorality and has no intention to change.
- If you entice others to sexual immorality (maybe in the back seat or back room), Jesus Himself has something against you!

Clearly, God *does* expect you to live according to His standard and not your own. In fact, as you just read in 1 Thessalonians 4:3, the Bible flatly states that this is God's will for your life. So take His command seriously and flee sexual immorality. Dump your own standards and choose freedom. You can, you know.

So why *don't* we choose to be pure? While our culture is thoroughly sensual to its core, it's not as though we're helpless victims of some vast conspiracy to ensnare us sexually. After all, Fred raised two sons and two daughters to adulthood smack dab in the middle of this culture, with them attending public schools, and they remained free.

From Steve: We Are Not Victims

Like Fred with his kids, I also raised a pure child—in my case in Laguna Beach, California, the heart of Orange County. Drugs, drinking, and sex were all a strong part of the school culture there, but my daughter made some excellent choices that set her apart. Before reaching high school, she had learned to say no and still feel good about herself, so by the time she graduated from Laguna Beach High School, she was one of a tiny minority who had never had a drink and had never smoked, taken a drug, or had sex. When it comes to saying no, she was a superstar, living proof that you don't have to be ruled by your culture, even today.

Clearly, while we *do* have a natural propensity to slip into sexual sin, we're not helpless victims here. The truth is, as men we've simply *chosen*, consciously or subconsciously, to mix in our own standards of sexual conduct with God's standard. Somewhere along the way, God's standard felt unnatural or too difficult, so we created a softer, gentler mixture—something new, something comfortable, something mediocre.

From Fred: Not Even a Hint

Now let's go one step deeper in defining our target on this battlefield:

Among you there must not be even a hint of sexual immorality. (Ephesians 5:3)

Given my promiscuous past, this verse was stunning to me. I murmured, *Man, a hint doesn't sound like much.* Well, it isn't.

Once I got serious about the battle, this scripture led me to inspect my life for any little hint of sexual immorality that might be tripping me up. I also wanted to put together the following list of what to avoid on my path to victory. Perhaps this list can help in your own inspection process:

- Do you tell off-color jokes? Do you use double entendres and coarse jesting?
- Do you surf the channels or internet hoping to catch a glimpse of something hot and racy?
- When a certain woman at your work calls in sick or absent, do you feel down a bit all day?
- If you're a manager, when you hired your last employee out of a pool of ten applicants, did you just happen to pick the prettiest one with the largest cup size?
- Do you lust over the lingerie ads in print or online?
- Are you regularly watching other people have sex in movies?
- Are you watching exercise shows and YouTube videos to get close-up views of women?
- Are you holding your gaze on joggers in nylon shorts and on curvy gym rats in their yoga pants?
- Do you look at cute girls walking and mutter to yourself, "Nice rear!"

- Are you flirting in ways that don't honor your wife or your God?
- Are you sexually fantasizing about the woman you're communicating with online?
- Are you fantasizing about another woman when you are in bed with your wife?
- Are you daydreaming about women other than your wife?
- Are you having hot, sexual dreams about other women at night?
- Are you thinking longingly and sexually about old girlfriends?
- Are you sometimes driving down the road thinking about that woman at work, even as your wife is riding with you?
- Are questions like these popping into your mind? *Does she ever think of me when she's not at work? What is she doing right now? Is she really happy with her husband?*
- Do you chafe and get angry about answering questions like these?

Many guys brush off this list as "little things" that don't really matter. I might have agreed, if not for God's direction in Ephesians 5:3. And then when I declared war on these "little" thoughts and actions and eliminated them from my life, a vast sexual pressure lifted from my life. Clearly, then, they aren't little things. If even one item from this list is evident in your life, you aren't avoiding every hint of sexual immorality. In fact, your purity standards are mixed.

Destruction and Loathing

A purity mixture can ensnare a man and destroy a people. When the Israelites entered the Promised Land, God told them to cross the Jordan River and destroy every evil thing in their new homeland. That meant killing all the heathen people and crushing their pagan gods. God warned them that if they failed to do this, their culture would "mix" with the pagan cultures and they would adopt depraved practices.

But the Israelites were not careful to destroy everything. They found it easier and easier to stop short as they tired of war. Besides, they soon noticed the beauty of the daughters of the land, so they pulled back from full obedience. In time, the things and the people left undestroyed became a snare to them, and in the end, the

Israelites became adulterous in their relationship to God and repeatedly turned their backs on Him.

As promised, the Lord removed them from their land. But just before the destruction of Jerusalem and the final deportation of her inhabitants, He prophesied this about His people in their coming captivity:

In the nations where they have been carried captive, those who escape will remember me—how I have been grieved by their adulterous hearts, which have turned away from me, and by their eyes, which have lusted after their idols. *They will loathe themselves for the evil they have done.* (Ezekiel 6:9)

When you entered the Promised Land of *your* salvation, you were told to eliminate every hint of sexual immorality in your life, lest it become a snare in your relationship with God. Since you've entered your land, have you failed to crush sexual sin? Every hint of it? If not, no matter how innocently it all began, you've likely come to the point of loathing yourself for that failure, just like the Israelites. If that's where you are, there's still hope, of course.

But you must declare war, and the mixing must stop. You must go God's way. We'll discuss what that looks like in the next chapter.

5

Obedience or Mere Excellence?

Why do we find it so easy to mix our standards regarding sexual sin and so difficult to firmly commit to purity? Because we've gotten used to it, for one thing. We easily tolerate mixed standards regarding our purity because we tolerate mixed standards in most other areas of life. Understanding the reason for this may be as simple as understanding one unique aspect of the male brain.

As much as you may have been told that men and women are alike in every fundamental way, we hope you realize how silly that notion is. Women aren't like men. Men aren't like women. The Bible tells us so, and modern science has proven it time and again. Significant brain differences between men and women lie at the root of these gender distinctions, and one of those differences explains why men so easily dilute God's standards.

First, a little background. English psychologist Simon Baron-Cohen explains the contrasts between male and female brains in his excellent book *The Essential Difference*. He writes that most men have "S-type" brains predominantly hardwired for understanding and building systems (including social systems), while women predominantly have "E-type" brains hardwired for empathy. Because of men's S-type brains, their place in their social hierarchy is of utmost priority to them. Left to their natural tendencies, they'll avoid *anything* that might drop their status with their peers, which explains why guys easily bail on their purity standards in the face of peer pressure. Baron-Cohen says it this way:

Women tend to value the development of altruistic, reciprocal relationships. Such relationships require good empathizing skills. In contrast, men tend to value power, politics, and competition. . . .

Boys are more likely than girls to endorse competitive items . . . and to rate social status as more important than intimacy. . . .

In a group, boys are quick to establish a "dominance hierarchy." . . .

The boys spend more time monitoring and maintaining the hierarchy. It seems to matter more to them. . . .

In the summer camp study . . . once a boy was put down [verbally] . . . *other* (lower-status) boys in the cabin jumped in to cement this victim's even-lower status. This was a means of establishing their own dominance over him. . . . Boys tend to be more often on the watch for opportunities to climb socially. . . .

The male social agenda is more *self-centered* in relation to the group, with all the benefits this can bring [like the best invitations and the best girls], and it protects one's status within this social system.[*]

From Fred: The Battle Starts When You're Young

While this material is quite enlightening on its face, I would like to flesh out these truths with a story from my early teens that perfectly illustrates how our S-type brains impact us in day-to-day life, especially in relation to every man's battle.

Believe it or not, my commitment to sexual purity was absolutely ironclad when I entered junior high, even though I wasn't yet committed to God. I had my own good reasons, though, because my parents had divorced when I was in fifth grade. Maybe I've lived worse years than that one, but I can't remember one. My mom's heart was shattered, and since my bedroom was next to hers, her anguished cries often seeped through the walls to awaken me at night. I'd slip into her room to console her, and sometimes she'd grab my hands and desperately search my eyes for

---

[*] Simon Baron-Cohen, *The Essential Difference: Male and Female Brains and the Truth About Autism* (New York: Basic Books, 2004), 32–33, 36–38, 41, 45.

forgiveness, her tormented apologies shattering my heart: "I'm so sorry I couldn't be the woman your dad wanted! I'm so sorry I can't be the father you're going to need and that you'll grow up without! I'm trying so hard to make up for it."

She'd fall back onto her bed in wrenching sobs, crying her eyes out. All I could do was sit there helpless, patting her arm in silent sympathy.

I despised my father in those moments. His selfish, miserable character. His pathetic mistresses in their wretched miniskirts and go-go boots. Night after cruel night, I'd swear with everything in me that I'd *never* treat women the way he did or *ever* use women for my sexual amusement. That vow was driven deeply into the bedrock of my soul by my mother's tears. It seemed unshakable, but of course, I'd not yet heard of or experienced the S-type male brain.

Two painful years passed. I entered seventh grade and strapped on the pads that autumn for my first year of tackle football. I was an overnight sensation, the undisputed star running back on the Linn-Mar Junior High football team in Marion, Iowa. I was suddenly planted squarely atop the social hierarchy as one of the "popular people." I was soon invited to the first elite party of the fall at Kathy Johnson's house. As I walked up her driveway that Friday night, I knew I had arrived, in more ways than one.

Still, I felt pretty nervous as I neared her house because I wasn't quite sure what went on at these things. As I entered the side door into the kitchen, I was thinking, *I hope there'll be a lot of laughing and goofing around with the guys.*

I felt a bit better when Kathy's parents welcomed me with open arms, but the calm faded quickly after Mr. Johnson shook my hand and pointed me toward the stairs leading to the rec room in the basement. "You go have some fun," he said. Then he winked.

What was that *all about?* I mused as I stepped through the basement door. The wink seemed creepy and unsettling. But I hadn't seen *anything* yet.

My foot had just hit the basement floor when a classmate named Janice leaped in front of me like a big tarantula. Now *that* was creepy!

You see, Janice had blossomed early up top, and as she slyly grinned and brushed her chest against me, my alarms started ringing. Nodding coyly toward the guest bedroom to her right, she purred, "Wanna play school? I'll be the teacher, and you can be my pet. I'll teach you everything you need to know. Good students really learn a lot in my class."

"Ah, I'm not so sure . . ."

I searched frantically over her shoulder for some way of escape, but the lights were too low to see much, and besides, whatever I *could* see was blowing my mind. My classmates were paired off on the couches or hunkered down in corners, and most of them were making out. I was shocked they'd be kissing in front of everybody. *What in the world?*

The tarantula demanded my attention once more. "Listen, if you try hard in my class, I'll give you an A," Janice teased.

Ugh. Janice wasn't going to give up easily on the chance to "school" me, and something told me that her first lesson plan would take us well beyond the elementary-level kissing I was seeing around the dim rec room. I hadn't even done *that* with a girl before, so I stalled for time. "Uh . . . uh . . . gee, Janice, I like Amy now," I stammered.

Just then, our host, Kathy, popped over to join our conversation. I'd *never* been so glad to see a girl in my life!

"Did you hear what Freddie just told me?" Janice announced to Kathy. "He likes Amy."

The pair looked at each other with Cheshire cat grins.

"Oh, you *do*," said Kathy. "I think we can do something about that, don't you, Janice?"

With that, the two girls disappeared. Sorely relieved to have dodged a major bullet, I was terribly embarrassed to tiptoe past several necking couples as I searched for an empty nook where I could disappear into the shadows. No such luck. Just as I was about to fade into the gloom with a deep sigh, the two girls found me, with Amy locked in their arms between them.

"Amy, Freddie just told us he likes you!" Janice announced with fanfare. Then she and Kathy vanished.

Oh, brother! I'm dead now!

I felt so naked! I had never even spoken to Amy before, and I knew she was way out of my league. In fact, she was out of *everyone's* league. Amy was the cutest girl at Linn-Mar, and everyone knew it, including me.

"Uh, hi, Amy," I began awkwardly. I tried to come up with something witty to say, but this social plebe couldn't think too fast under the gun. "How are you doing?" *Okay, I'm the biggest dork this side of the Rockies,* I thought, groaning inside.

"I'm fine," Amy said, shifting her feet restlessly.

An uncomfortable silence fell. I looked at my feet and said, "Listen, I'm not—"

"Don't worry about it," Amy replied.

It was getting hot. "I'm going to see if there's anything to eat," I blurted foolishly.

My face burned with humiliation as I walked up the stairs. After nibbling on a carrot and a piece of cheese, I slipped out the side door while no one was looking, demoralized and feeling like an idiot. I didn't like that feeling, and in the short time it took me to cover the six blocks home and slip the key into the lock, something had changed in me.

Before that night at Kathy Johnson's party, I was thinking for myself and defending my standards. Sure, I was young, but I'd carefully considered how I planned to treat women during my life. My mom's pain had taught me right from wrong, and like any real man, I intended to protect the women around me by living right no matter what anybody else thought. That's what men do, or so I thought when I was in seventh grade.

On the way home from the party, however, I discovered something else men do as a result of their S-type brains. Other voices began speaking up on the matter in my head, pressing me to adjust my thinking. By the time I got home and flipped on the kitchen lights, I looked a little less like me and a little more like them. I'd stepped toward the group and my place in the group and away from who I'd always been.

My vow to treat girls with respect and tenderness didn't look so important anymore. While I avoided parties (and tarantulas) for quite some time, I was clearly drifting from my original, thoughtful stance on how I would treat girls.

One painful social event at Kathy's house was all it took to rock my standards loose. Only one.

A Turn Toward the Crowd

Decades later, it's still hard to believe what happened that night. After all, I hated the way my dad used women. Why did I sell out so easily after one measly party? Well, that's the natural impact of the male S-type brain. By nature, if guys aren't aware of this trait, they will often do *anything* to protect their place in the social order. If you don't respect this vulnerability and properly defend it, your standards will slide toward that mushy middle ground every time.

Make no mistake—you *can* defend it. Had someone explained how my brain was structured, I would have seen my churning pain for what it was: a false pressure ginned up by my S-type brain, well outside my conscious will. Had I known how I was naturally wired, I could have chosen to ignore it.

Instead, my social-climbing brain let position and rank dominate my thinking even though Mom's pain had cast a hero's heart inside me. Only this can explain why a young star running back at the top of his game would sell out his standards at the first sign of social trouble. I couldn't have cared less about kissing some girl when the evening began, but as I scurried home that evening, my male, S-type brain was screaming, *Listen up! Your place is slipping with the gang!* Before long, being me and being honorable no longer meant the same thing.

It's this unique brain structure that gets us used to diluting God's standards in every area of life, because this kind of social pressure isn't exerted by just a few friends from time to time at Friday night parties. The pressure to mix our standards and fit in nicely with the group is exerted *constantly* by our entire culture. And because of this vulnerability in our brains, we are quick to stop short of God's call to ease our way in social situations. We end up valuing what's around us in the *world* far more than we value the *Word.* I see that reflected everywhere I go because the male brain is the same everywhere I go.

Does our vulnerability to social and cultural pressure mean that we can ignore Scripture? Does God give Christian men a pass on His standards if following them would put our status at risk? Or does the Lord expect us to live differently from those around us, in true obedience to His Word, whatever the social cost?

Answer these questions wrong and you imperil your development as a child of

God. It won't change your status as a family member, of course. Every Christian child—everyone "born again"—has his Father's DNA. But only the *mature* child has his Father's *character*. Learning to think and act like Him no matter how it affects our spots on the social ladder is what Christianity is all about. But mixing in our own cultural beliefs—the human way of thinking—will abort this maturation process in our lives.

If you desire sexual freedom, you can't mix God's standards with the standards of our sex-saturated culture. Consider what the common cultural mind-set says to men:

- Hey, looking and lusting is just guys being guys, having a little fun.
- God wouldn't have made women this beautiful if He didn't want us to look at them. After all, appreciating women is no different than going to a museum to appreciate fine art.
- Porn and masturbation are nothing more than useful pressure releases.
- Why worry about what I look at? Jesus's blood covers it all anyway. I won't go to hell! I'm forgiven.
- Porn is just pictures on paper. Nothing I do in the privacy of my home hurts anyone.

As long as you believe *any* of these things from the secular mind-set, you'll never be pure. Ever.

Some time ago, I was in Costa Rica to record a *Focus on the Family* radio broadcast with Focus's Latin arm. My broadcast host told me that they had just released their survey of three hundred evangelical Christian men in Costa Rica that very day. Since it was applicable to our broadcast, he also shared with me one of the questions on the survey, the one asking whether these married men had ever had a sexual affair outside marriage. Two hundred ninety-nine said yes! Nothing but mixture there.

My host explained that adultery had always been tacitly approved in the Costa Rican culture, so Christian men there lived a mixed standard. They commonly had sex outside marriage in spite of biblical mandates.

I couldn't believe the survey results. Only one man out of three hundred stayed true to the fixed biblical principles? In my mind, such a ridiculous and senseless level of mixture can be explained only by the male S-type brain and its absolute, subconscious focus upon fitting in with the local culture. That same brain science explains the rampant justification among American Christians and other believers who excuse their illicit sexual behavior and hold casual attitudes toward sexual sin.

That isn't how it is supposed to be in the kingdom of God. When Jesus called His twelve disciples into service, He could have given them any title. But He chose to call them apostles, and He did so because of the message the name conveyed at the time. In those days, Roman legions would sweep through and take down powerful cities before moving on to the next one. Too often, they found that when they returned to these conquered cities, they would have to retake them in battle because nothing had been done to lock their victories in place the first time through.

So the Romans developed a new kind of military leader called an *apostolos*. The job of this general was to move in after the battle was over to replace the existing local culture with his own Roman culture, including his art, sculpture, and music. By the leader's putting in place a new way of life, the conquered people would begin to think and act like Romans and would be far less likely to rebel against their conquerors' rule.

While it's true that Jesus may have used the term *apostolos* because its most common meaning at the time was "sent one," I personally believe that Jesus christened His disciples "apostles" to convey a message related to the word's military context. After all, it was never His intent to merely mix His ways in with the rotting cultural soup of the local peoples of this earth, just to freshen or sweeten their pot a bit. No, He had won His war and was now sending in His *apostolos* to lock down His victory at the cultural level. He intended to flip over the pots altogether and pour out His own living recipe to fill them, His kingdom culture wholly replacing the godless cultures.

But as is evident from the statistics about porn use and infidelity within the church, in America and around the world, few of our brothers in Christ are doing what Jesus hoped they'd do. Instead, biblical standards are being rejected in favor of cultural norms. It's not even seen as an issue. It's all normal, right, and true because it's common. Everyone thinks this way, so that's how the Christians roll too. The common is comfortable.

Perhaps the culture around you is driving your thinking as well. Maybe you're one of those Christians who regularly peek into other people's bedrooms to watch couples having sex, for instance. Of course, we call it going to the movies. While eating popcorn and sitting in the same theater with dozens of others may make things seemlier, the truth of the matter is that in America it's normal, right, and true for Christians to be Peeping Toms.

Oh, I know. It's common, and perhaps everyone *does* think this way. But it's still mixture. It's still stopping short at a false finish line.

Most of all, it's still devastating and disastrous to sexual purity. As you might expect, Jesus isn't all that interested in your social comfort or your status with your peers. He's after your character, and He's after complete cultural change. So let's close this chapter by inspecting your current approach to God's standards and the social circles you run in.

Excellence or Obedience?

What is your aim in life—excellence or obedience? What's the difference? To aim for obedience is to aim for perfection and not for excellence, which is actually something less. Your answer to this question reveals whether your spirit or your status-focused male brain is doing your thinking for you.

Your answer also discloses which culture owns your heart: Christ's kingdom culture or the worldly one.

"Wait a minute!" you reply. "I thought excellence and perfection were the same thing."

Sometimes they appear to be. But the truth is, in most arenas, excellence is a mixed standard, not a fixed standard.

Let us show you what we mean. American businesses are in search of excellence. They *could* be in search of perfection, of course—perfect products, perfect service— but perfection is too costly and eats into profits. Businesses know that rather than be perfect, it's enough to *seem* perfect to their customers. By stopping short of perfection, they find a profitable balance between quality and costs. To find this balance, they often look to their competitors to discover the best practices of their industry: *How far can we go and still seem perfect? How far can we stop short and still be considered a good business?*

Now let's shift to our churches. Rather than search the Word for best practices, Christians often use each other as benchmarks, much as businesses do: *How far can I go and still be considered a good Christian?* When you ask this question, you're looking for a middle ground where you can find a profitable balance between a seemingly quality Christian life and the social costs of being too perfect or too different.

But is it ever truly profitable for Christians to stop short at this middle ground of excellence? You know, that place where social costs are low and you can live balanced somewhere between paganism and obedience? The answer: *Never!* Sure, in business it may be profitable to *seem* perfect, but in the *spiritual* realm, it's only *comfortable* to seem perfect. It is never profitable spiritually.

Clearly, then, excellence isn't the same as obedience or perfection. In the Christian life, the search for mere excellence leaves us overwhelmingly vulnerable to snare after snare since it allows room for mixture of our ways with God's ways. The search for obedience does not leave us such room. As Christ followers, we must shoot for the fixed standard of obedience if we're to ever find sexual freedom. We must get comfortable with being different.

From Fred: Asking the Wrong Question

I was the perfect example of someone who wasn't shooting for God's fixed standard of obedience. I was teaching classes at church, chairing activity groups there, and attending discipleship training. My church attendance was exemplary, and I spoke the Christian language. Like a businessman seeking the best business practices, I was comparing myself against the other men at church, asking, *How far can I go and still be called a Christian?* That was enough for me at first.

But that is never enough for God because He doesn't want His children to have just His DNA; He wants us to have His character too. I would've never developed His character by hanging around that middle ground, pondering, *How far can I go and still look Christian enough?* To reach maturity, I needed to be asking a different question: *How holy can I be?*

Let me use a story to demonstrate once more the difference between excellence and obedience. Pete and Mary attended my premarriage class, and Pete impressed me from day one. He lapped up anything I said, nodding in assent at even the most difficult teachings regarding the husband's responsibilities, such as servanthood.

At the end of the seventh week, Pete and Mary stopped me after class. "Your discussion on sexual purity really hit home last week," Pete began, "especially when you said that viewing pornography and X-rated movies won't strengthen your sex life. My first wife used to rent X-rated movies for me, and we would watch them together before going to bed. In the end, it hurt us." Then he added, "Mary and I will not do this in our marriage."

Sounds impressive. But had Pete stepped into true obedience, or by ruling out pornography and X-rated movies, had he stopped short at mere excellence?

The answer came when Mary joined the conversation. "We've been having an ongoing struggle over what we watch together. We'll often stream a movie to watch at my apartment, but you know how it is. Most of the popular movies have some pretty racy scenes, and I'm feeling more and more uncomfortable with all that. When it gets steamy, I tell Pete we need to turn it off, but he gets angry, arguing that we're paying good money for it. So I go into the kitchen to do some work while he finishes watching."

She got a tear in her eye and looked down. "I don't feel these movies are good for us," she said. "I've asked him to stop for my sake, but he won't. We make it a practice to pray together before he goes home. But after these movies, I often feel dirty and cheap, and our prayer feels strange. I feel these movies are coming between us as a couple and also between us and God."

Of course, Pete was embarrassed. He'd been caught stopping short at a false middle ground. Whether consciously or subconsciously, he'd judged by the mixed standards of his peers that he could watch popular movies with racy sexual situations and still "seem" Christian enough at church without having to pay the full cost of true obedience. Up until that moment, that was all he'd needed to know.

To his credit, though, Pete asked me what he should do. I told him to follow Mary's lead and not watch the sexy films, and he agreed to do so.

Excellence is deceptive. It helps us sound good and comfortably fit in with the crowd rather than pay the price of true obedience. Too often there's no challenging voice like Mary's calling us to obedience and perfection. All we hear is our culture and the voices of our friends on the social ladders around us, and those voices never call us higher. Satisfied with mere excellence and desiring to fit in, we stop short of God's standards and mix in some of our own. We move nearer to our peers only to find distance from God.

In so many areas, we're often sitting together on the middle ground of excellence, a good distance from God. When challenged by His higher standards, our S-type brains take over subconsciously behind the scenes. We're comforted that we don't look too different from those around us. Trouble is, we don't look much different from non-Christians either.

Have we gone blind? What can we expect from our across-the-board commitment to the middle ground?

The Right Response

Israel's King Josiah was only twenty-six years of age when in *his* culture he faced a similar situation of neglect for God's standards. In 2 Chronicles 34, we read how a copy of God's Law—long forgotten—had been found during a large-scale renovation of the temple. Then Josiah listened as the Law was read aloud to him, bringing inescapably to his attention God's standards and the people's failure to live up to them.

Josiah didn't say, "Oh, come on, we've lived this way for years. Let's not get legalistic about all this!" No, he was horrified. He tore his robes as a sign of grief and despair. "Great is the LORD's anger" (verse 21), he said as he immediately acknowledged his people's negligence and sought God's further guidance.

God quickly answered with these words about Josiah's reaction:

Because your heart was responsive and you humbled yourself before God when you heard what he spoke against this place and its people, and because you humbled yourself before me and tore your robes and wept in my presence, I have heard you, declares the LORD. (verse 27)

Notice how, at this point, Josiah immediately led the entire nation in a thorough return to obedience to God's standards:

Then the king . . . went up to the temple of the LORD with the people of Judah, the inhabitants of Jerusalem, the priests and the Levites—all the people from the least to the greatest. He read in their hearing all the words of the Book of the Covenant, which had been found in the temple of the LORD. The king stood by his pillar and renewed the covenant in the presence of the LORD—to follow the LORD and keep his commands, statutes and decrees with all his heart and all his soul, and to obey the words of the covenant written in this book.

Then he had everyone in Jerusalem and Benjamin pledge themselves to it; the people of Jerusalem did this in accordance with the covenant of God, the God of their ancestors.

Josiah removed all the detestable idols from all the territory belonging to the Israelites, and he had all who were present in Israel serve the LORD their God. As long as he lived, they did not fail to follow the LORD, the God of their ancestors. (verses 29–33)

No mixture there. Knowing that God's standard is the standard of true life, Josiah rose up and tore down everything that was in opposition to God. In a sense, he was playing the *apostolos* role in his kingdom, dumping the old culture entirely and establishing God's culture in its place.

Counting the Cost

What about you? Obviously, you don't have the position or authority to change the entire culture of your country like Josiah did, but you can still play that *apostolos* role in your work situation, your marriage, your family, and perhaps your immediate social hierarchy. You can even transform the culture of your local church.

Now that you've listened to God's Word and comprehend His standard of sexual purity, will you be responsive and humble yourself before God like Josiah did? Are you willing to make a covenant to hold to that standard with all your heart and soul? Will you tear down every hint of sexual immorality that stands in opposition to God?

Sexual impurity has become rampant in the church because, as individuals, we've ignored the costly work of obedience to God's standards.

If you don't kill every hint of immorality—even those that are common—you'll be captured by your tendency as a male to draw sexual gratification and chemical highs through your eyes, and your mixed standards will play right into the Enemy's hands.

But you can't deal with your male eyes until you first deal with your S-type brain and reject your right to mix your standards. As you ask, "How holy can I be?" you must pray and commit to a new relationship with God, fully aligned with His ways and His call to obedience.

6

Just by Being Male

O ur very maleness represents the primary reason for the pervasiveness of sexual impurity among men. We said it earlier, but we want to say it again: in a very real sense, by nature we are set up to fall into sexual sin.

We've just explored one aspect of our maleness—our S-type brains—and we've seen how it leads us to stop short of God's standards. But the effects of our maleness don't stop there, not by a long shot. Let's delve into yet another even more calamitous vulnerability in our male nature that leaves us heavily exposed to sexual sin.

From Fred: Our Very Maleness

Before I even knew that my wife, Brenda, was pregnant with our fourth child, I became convinced through prayer that our future child would be a boy—our second son. I was so convinced of this that, during Brenda's pregnancy, I told this to her and a few close friends. (Brenda did have ultrasound tests, but we asked our doctor and technicians not to tell us the baby's gender.)

As delivery day neared, the pressure rose. "Why did I tell everyone?" I whined. "What if it's a girl? What if I'm wrong? I'll look like an idiot!"

With the start of Brenda's labor pains, the pressure on me seemed to double every minute. Finally, standing under the bright lights of the delivery room and watching a little head crowning toward birth, I knew the moment of truth was near.

The baby came out faceup. *Good,* I thought. *I'll have a perfect view.* The shoulders emerged. *Just a few more inches,* I thought. And then? *Auugh! What are you doing, Doctor?* He turned the baby toward himself at the last moment, just as the hips and legs popped out. Now I could see only the baby's back. *C'mon, c'mon,* I cried out inside.

Maddeningly, the doctor and nurse said nothing. Methodically and efficiently, they dried the baby, suctioned the baby's throat, and slapped a silly little cap on him or her. When the doctor finally presented our new child to me, the legs were flopping apart. Immediately looking down, I just had to know.

"It's a boy!" I exclaimed.

Michael is now twenty-seven and his older brother, Jasen, is thirty-five, and I can assure you that they are both definitely males. As I raised them, I was aware of the natural attributes inherent to maleness that would touch every aspect of their battles for sexual purity, just as these same characteristics affected me.

My insights helped them immensely on the battlefield because maleness matters, and nowhere does our maleness matter more than in our eyes.

Males Receive Sexual Gratification Through the Eyes

Our eyes give us guys the means to sin broadly and at will. We don't need a date or a mistress. We don't need to wait for a woman to drop by our apartment. We have our eyes to call upon, and we can draw genuine sexual gratification through them at any time. We're turned on by female curves and nudity in any way, shape, or form.

We aren't picky. It can come in a sensual, serpentine dance scene from the voluptuous Beyoncé or in a photograph of a nude, nameless stranger just as easily as in a romantic interlude with one's wife. We have a visual ignition switch when it comes to viewing the female anatomy.

Women seldom understand this because they aren't sexually stimulated in the same way and haven't personally experienced what the eyes can do in the way we have. Their ignitions are tied to touch and relationship, which to them seems nobler and more virtuous. As a result, they often view this visual aspect of our sexuality as shallow and dirty, even detestable. Any effort from a husband to put a positive spin on this "vision factor" by suggesting that his wife use it to her advantage in the bedroom may be met with disdainful scorn. For instance, upon hearing such a suggestion from me (Fred), Brenda spat haughtily, "So I suppose I have to buy some cheap teddy and prance around like a saloon girl!"

Somehow, I laughed at the time! But visual sexual gratification is no laughing matter in your fight for sexual purity. Given what the sight of nudity does to the pleasure centers of our brains—and these days it's pretty easy to see many naked or near-naked women—it's no wonder our eyes and minds resist control.

From Fred: A Favorite Moment in Time

My favorite moment of the past two decades in the debate surrounding pornography took place in the chambers of the United States Senate when Senator Sam Brownback of Kansas introduced a congressional hearing on whether pornography should continue to be protected as a form of free speech or whether it should instead be regulated like other toxic and addictive drugs. Interesting question!

Regulated like drugs? But I thought pornography was nothing more than pictures on paper or pixels on a screen. Viewing porn is just guys being guys! The average man would react in this exact way, and why not? Porn use is commonplace, and viewing it is considered normal behavior. Isn't this the way everyone thinks?

But experts on pornography's effects on brain chemistry would disagree, and they testified in those Senate hearings that it was time to quit regarding porn as just another form of artistic expression. When it was his turn to share, Dr. Jeffrey Satinover made one of the most vivid, concise, and powerful statements I've ever heard regarding porn's impact upon the brain:

> Modern science allows us to understand that the underlying nature of an
> addiction to pornography is chemically nearly identical to a heroin addiction:
> Only the delivery system is different, and the sequence of steps.[*]

---

[*] Jeffrey Satinover, MS, MD, "U.S. Senate Hearing Testimony on Pornography Part 4," Oxbow Academy, November 17, 2004, https://oxbowacademy.net/educationalarticles/senate_hearing_porn4.

Stop for a moment and let that sink in. The eye, when viewing porn, is like a needle full of heroin being injected into the bloodstream.

Really? Like heroin? Come on, Fred!

When you look at the science, it simply isn't hyperbole or an overstatement. Granted, the impact of porn is not as physically harsh as with heroin itself. I'm not going to find you strung out in the corner of some rat-infested warehouse or sitting in a Walmart parking lot passed out at the steering wheel, with your kids strapped into their car seats, just because you flipped through several popular porn sites on your smartphone. But porn's chemistry inside a male's body is *extremely* powerful and creates a significant dependency, both physically and emotionally.

I can also tell you that one of the most dangerous things you can do in your battle for purity is to laugh this off and underestimate the addictive impact of the sexual gratification you draw through your eyes. As long as you continue selling this truth short, you will continue to lose on the battlefield because you won't be giving your eyes the proper defense and protection.

The University of Pennsylvania's Dr. Mary Anne Layden is perhaps America's leading researcher into porn's impact upon the brain, and she was invited to speak to our senators too. Perhaps you recall Steve saying that men receive a chemical high from sexually charged images and that part of the chemistry is the secretion of epinephrine into the bloodstream, locking into the brain a picture of the sensuality you're viewing.

Dr. Layden discussed this exact process when she said, "That image is in your brain forever. If that was an addictive substance, you, at any point for the rest of your life, could in a nanosecond draw it up [and get high]."[*]

Any honest man knows this is true from his own experience, and if he's even *more* honest, he knows he doesn't need today's tsunami of digital technology on his smartphone to freeze these tantalizing images of the female form into his brain. All he needs is to take a casual stroll through a mall. I was reminded of this around sixteen years ago after my son Michael returned from a shopping trip with Brenda and his two sisters. They returned lugging large, lumpy shopping bags. From my

---

[*] Stuart Shepard, "Porn Is Like Heroin in the Brain," Focus on the Family, November 19, 2004, www.freerepublic .com/focus/news/1284238/posts?page=92.

basement office, I could hear them making a ruckus upstairs as they came in from the garage. Suddenly, everything went quiet. I knew the girls must have run up to their room on the second floor to put away their new treasures.

I returned my focus to the computer and wouldn't find out what ensued until later. What happened is that Michael—eleven years old at the time—snuck up behind his mom in the kitchen and wrapped his short arms around Brenda's waist. My wife turned around with a smile, thinking he was thanking her for a fun time at the mall.

"I love you too, Michael!" she said as she bent down to him with a bright smile of affection.

But my youngest son wasn't smiling. Instead, she discovered a pair of searching eyes leveled upon hers like lasers. "Mom, how do you get pictures of women in their underwear out of your head?" he implored.

Brenda, to her credit, kept smiling, but inside she wondered if she had heard her son correctly. When she realized she had, she didn't miss a beat.

"I think that's a great question for your dad," she said, tousling his hair and pointing him toward the basement. "But before you go, exactly what kind of pictures are you talking about?"

"Remember when we walked to the food court today?"

"Sure."

"Well, when we walked past that 'secret store,' I looked at those women wearing that underwear. I haven't been able to get those pictures out of my head all day."

Suddenly, everything clicked for Brenda—and for me when Michael told me what had happened. That "secret store" was Victoria's Secret, the intimate-apparel emporium with lifelike mannequins in suggestive poses and wearing frilly lingerie. Perhaps consciously for the first time, Michael had experienced the ability of male eyes to chemically lock in such sensual images with only a glance.

Now, add Michael's story to the two comments from Dr. Satinover and Dr. Layden before the Senate. What do these three examples tell us about men and their sexuality?

First, God created men this way and there is no reason to attach shame to a man's visual nature. This aspect of our sexuality is not shallow or dirty; it is simply male.

Second, if a man falls into sexual sin, it's not necessarily a reflection of his spiritual life, at least not at first. Consider Michael, for instance. At the time, Michael was one of the most spiritual preadolescents I'd ever met. He later developed a deep passion for prayer and worship during his teen years and became one of the most spiritual young men I know. Those images didn't get locked into his brain because he was spiritually deficient as a boy.

On top of that, Michael wasn't even interested in girls when he was eleven years old. As they say in Iowa, he wouldn't have known a girl from a bale of hay at the time, so he wasn't looking into that "secret store" window in an attempt to lust. He was just minding his own business and happened to glance up into the display window as he meandered to lunch with his mom and sisters.

The fact that these images locked into his brain was not a reflection of his spirituality but rather a reflection of his maleness. His eyes were merely doing what they were created to do. I've heard men cry out, "I'm a Christian! Why can't I stop this sexual sin? Shouldn't I be more spiritual?" I'm hoping you can see that a major part of the problem has more to do with how we are made than with how spiritual we are. The truth is, while this battle for purity has spiritual components, it is actually a lot more physical in scope than most men realize. Beating yourself up for "not being spiritual enough" is far too simplistic and not helpful. For most guys, the battle is not so much about guarding the heart as it is about guarding the eyes.

An Inconvenient Truth

Another key truth about our visual nature is that the male eye can perform sexual foreplay, all on its own. That's right. Without even touching a woman.

We normally think of sexual foreplay as tactile or physical, like caressing or kissing a breast. But foreplay is any sensual action that naturally prepares the body for intercourse, that ignites passion, rocketing us by stages until we want to go all the way. It needn't be tactile.

So, what acts constitute foreplay? Certainly, mutual stroking of the genitals is foreplay. Even stroking the top of the thigh can be foreplay. (Young men may not see it that way, but fathers do! If you saw a boy stroking your daughter's thigh, I would bet that you wouldn't just wink and turn away.) When a girl lays her head in the lap of a teenage boy, that's foreplay—a mild form, perhaps, but that'll get his motor running at levels too high for young motors. Slow dancing can be foreplay if certain parts of the body are in close contact.

If you're married, you may be asking, *What does all this have to do with me? My foreplay happens only with my wife.*

Are you sure? Impurity of the eyes provides definite sexual gratification. Isn't that foreplay? When you see a hot movie scene, is there a twitch below your belt? What are you thinking when you're on the beach and suddenly meet a jaw-dropping beauty in a thong bikini? You gasp while Mission Control announces, "We have ignition!" You have her in bed on the spot, though only in your mind. Or you file away the image and fantasize about her later.

You stare at a sexy model and lust; you stare some more and lust some more. Your motor revs into the red zone, and you need some type of release or the engine's going to blow. You have an erection and your body is ready for intercourse, though you haven't even touched a woman. The work of your eyes is the only foreplay involved. Before long, you're masturbating.

No doubt about it: for men, visual sexual gratification is a form of sexual foreplay. A young husband named Alex remembers the time he was watching TV with his sister-in-law. The rest of the family was at the mall. "She was lying flat on her stomach on the floor in front of me, wearing tight shorts, and she'd fallen asleep watching TV. I was on the chair, and I happened to look down and see her upper thigh and a trace of her underwear. I tried to ignore it, but my heart started racing a little, and my eyes kept looking at her. It got so exciting that I began to stare and really lust. I had to release the pressure somehow, so I masturbated while she slept, right out in the open."

Note that the sexual gratification drawn through the eyes was real and genuine enough to prepare Alex's body for intercourse with only his eyes without even touching a woman. It's critical to recognize visual sexual impurity as foreplay. If viewing sensual things merely provides a flutter of appreciation for a woman's beauty, it is no different than viewing the awesome power of a thunderstorm racing over the Iowa cornfields. No sin. No problem.

But if it *is* foreplay, and if we're getting sexual gratification, what position does this put us in as men? Well, consider that half of all young people catch their first glimpse of porn before the age of thirteen.[*]

We expect that average age to fall even further as kids get their first iPad or tablet computer at younger ages. In many elementary school classrooms today, every child has his or her own iPad, and kids have a way of getting around adult controls.

The point is that we often get drawn into sexual sin long before we even recognize the dangers. As men, we are vulnerable because of our created nature. This also means that if we fathers are maintaining silence on this topic, we are likely dooming our sons to disaster. Think about it. What would have happened next for my Michael if I hadn't been at home, engaged, and ready to answer his question when Brenda sent him down to the basement to talk with me?

It's easy enough to figure out. The next time he went to the mall, Michael might have looked into another store window with scantily clad mannequins and found that something similar happened. Or he might have stumbled upon a movie or television show and found images locking into his brain there too. Pretty soon his curiosity would have led him to the family computer or an iPad, searches would have led to images of nude women, and before he knew it, his eyes would have become heat-seeking rockets like mine once were.

Thankfully, I helped Michael sort out his interesting afternoon at the mall. But for other boys, what if a father isn't there or is too scared to bring up the topic because he isn't sexually pure himself? Every young man's battlefield has been dramatically altered by sexual nuclear blasts from the internet and pornographic carpet bombing from cell phones, which have shelled his landscape beyond recognition. Early exposure is practically a given these days.

But that doesn't mean our young men *must* fall into a decade or two of losses before finally finding freedom, if ever. The truth is, guys can learn to defend themselves early so losses don't have to happen. Learning to control one's sexuality is just part of becoming a man, and young guys like Michael simply need someone to

---

[*] Danny Huerta, MSW, LCSW, LSSW, "Kids Viewing Porn—How Pervasive Is It?," Focus on the Family, 2018, www.focusonthefamily.com/parenting/sexuality/kids-and-pornography/kids-viewing-porn-how-pervasive-is-it.

teach them what is normal, right, and true and how to manage their eyes and their sex drives. There's no reason to bring shame into this picture. Everyone needs to be taught sometime.

And that goes for you too, whatever your age. *Every Man's Battle* will give you that knowledge, and if you have a son who needs you to pass on this knowledge, you'll find help in our book *Preparing Your Son for Every Man's Battle.* Engage with him, especially in those critical years between the ages of ten and thirteen. He'll need your insight badly.

The Plastic Brain

As we've said, our innate male design—particularly our visual nature—helps explain the prevalence of sexual sin among Christian guys. If you're ever going to learn how to manage your sexuality properly, you'll obviously need to guard your eyes effectively. If you don't control your eyes, they'll keep building pathways to your brain and flooding it with addictive pleasure chemicals.

Let's talk about these brain pathways for a moment. There's been a tremendous revolution in our understanding of the human brain over the last twenty years, especially in terms of its underlying structure. Your brain is nowhere near as static and inflexible as once believed. Instead, the brain is so "plastic" and malleable that even your personal behaviors and actions, including your porn use and masturbation, can literally mold and shape the underlying wiring of your brain—its neural pathways—and trap you more deeply into sin the longer you're involved. Clearly, your neuroplastic brain (and your ability to change your neural pathways through your choices) will impact purity's battlefield in a big way, both good and bad.

Perhaps a brief human biology lesson would be a good idea here. First of all, the brain is composed primarily of neurons, which are specialized cells that transmit electrical impulses, allowing the brain to do its work. The connections that bridge the gaps between the neurons and provide the cohesive electrical gridwork of communication are called synapses.

Synapses are not hard electrical connections between two neurons, like an Ethernet cord connecting your desktop computer to the internet. Instead, a synapse is more like a microscopic bit of fluidic space *between* the neurons, through which the electrical impulses "float" neurochemically from one side to the other.

Synapses require regular use for their very existence, and they are responsible for your brain's plasticity. For instance, when you take up a new activity and repeat a particular action again and again over time, the brain rewires itself by creating neural pathways (neurons connected by synapses and working together) to handle the impulses of that particular activity in speedier and more efficient fashion. This rewiring actually takes place in the synapses themselves, where the number of connections between the neurons are increased and strengthened by use, much like the muscle fibers in your triceps are increased and strengthened by doing daily push-ups.

On the other hand, if you ever stop a new activity and no longer use these connections, the synapses in that neural pathway weaken and eventually break down and die. The entire neuroplastic process is ruled by the use-it-or-lose-it principle, along with this catchy one: "Neurons that fire together wire together."

When masses of neurons fire in concert repeatedly—like when you're playing the piano—synaptic changes occur that powerfully connect large groups of neurons into neural maps that transport impulses faster and more efficiently through the brain. When necessary, new neural real estate is claimed by these new activities, again based on the level of use.

Let me (Fred) paint a clearer picture of this process for you. If you had performed exhaustive cranial research on Brenda three years ago, you wouldn't have found a trace of neural real estate assigned to playing the piano. But if you scanned her brain today after her having two years of daily practice, you'd discover that a considerable block of neural acreage has been annexed by her burgeoning piano skills, and a healthy, complex map of synaptic connections is flourishing to process it all.

Brenda indirectly controls the entire process. She sustains these synapses by practicing the piano; in this way, the synapses survive and thrive. If she ever gives up playing the piano, these same synaptic maps will fade, and her skills will eventually decompose and die. While every bit of the neurochemical and structural changes happens at the subconscious level, outside Brenda's awareness, she still has genuine life-or-death control over these neural pathways.

This neurological process is incredible, when you think about it. Based on your conscious decisions regarding your daily behavior and experiences, you can either bolster your synapses or allow them to languish. In other words, you have control over your neural pathways, which is extraordinarily useful in your battle for purity. I'll come back to this shortly.

From Fred: A Little Closer to Home

To illustrate this concept further, let's move from the piano to pornography. Recently, I counseled Ethan regarding his porn viewing and masturbation, including one particularly stubborn habit that occurred every Monday at noon, when his wife, Sophia, was out of the apartment working and he was home on his day off, handling child-care duties for their toddler daughter, Skylar. Every time the clock struck noon and he put his daughter down for a nap, he felt as though a demon wrapped a shepherd's hook around his neck and yanked him to the computer for a session of cyberporn and masturbation. The draw was overwhelming, and he just couldn't stop.

How did Ethan's habit become so mulish and tenacious that he could practically set his watch to the onset of temptation during Skylar's naptime? The answer is simple: Ethan had extensively rewired the neural pathways to his sexual pleasure centers through behavioral repetition at his computer screen every Monday at noontime.

With each session and each orgasm, the pleasure-giving neurotransmitter dopamine surged through Ethan's brain and lit up his pleasure centers. But dopamine also stimulates neuroplastic change, so that same surge of dopamine that thrilled Ethan also strengthened the synapses and consolidated the neural connections in his sexual maps. Newly enlarged and strengthened, the maps associated with his actions could now efficiently push him into future incidents of porn and masturbation, especially on Mondays at noon.

You see, dopamine also helps to lay down memories in your brain so that the next time you're in the same place at the same time, the brain remembers where to turn to be gratified again. In Ethan's case, his brain had determined exactly what Monday's noon naptime meant for his sexual pleasure centers and had learned how to push forcibly to get what it wanted.

Reprogram Your Brain?

Can Ethan's brain unlearn what it knows related to Skylar's naptime? Can Ethan ever kill his weekly habit? Well, let's go back to what you just read a short while ago. You have indirect control over your neuroplastic processes. Based upon your conscious decisions regarding your daily behavior and experiences, you can either bolster your synapses or allow them to languish. In other words, you have control over your neural pathways, which is extraordinarily useful in your battle for purity.

Ethan had the same indirect control that we all have, and he broke his habit through a set of consistent, conscious decisions. Before I share the details, let me paint a word picture about trains and railroads to help you understand how you can *unlearn* neuroplastic change through the use-it-or-lose-it principle.

About thirty miles north of my home, you'll find a set of rails over which 150 hoppers full of coal pass every half hour or so on their way to the East Coast from Wyoming. The tracks are so heavily used and so well maintained that you'd be hard pressed to find a weed or even a blade of grass between the rails if you cared to look. Dozens of locomotive engines fly over those tracks every single day, twice an hour, and nothing stands in the way to slow them down.

When I think of Ethan's neural pathways spanning his sexual maps, I think of those strong, efficient train tracks that stretch out as clean as a whistle. Ethan's sexual impulses could race over his tracks at will (especially on Mondays at noon) because nothing stood in the way of his powerful sexual engines.

But have you ever seen a set of abandoned tracks—lonely, overgrown, and rusting in the rain? With weeds and scrub brush growing past your ankles and even waist high between the rails and with thick saplings sinking their roots between the ties, those tracks have deteriorated to such a state that no hopper of coal could pass without derailing.

To unlearn the changes brought into your life by your corrupted neural pathways, you must abandon them in this same way. According to the use-it-or-lose-it principle, you must stop using them so that the synaptic connections will weaken, decompose, and die. When that happens, those once-smooth neural rails will become impossibly overgrown.

That's exactly what I helped Ethan to do. He had to stop reinforcing the neural pathways. He had to make Monday at noon mean something else entirely to his brain, and he did this by consistently changing what happened Monday at noon.

To put Ethan on the path to purity, I had him make a long list of things that he could do around the apartment after placing Skylar in her crib for a nap. He came up with fifty items. After laying her down, he'd take that list and choose three or four things to do over the next hour that would help him keep his mind off the computer. The tasks were fairly routine: washing the dishes, vacuuming the apartment, listening to a podcast sermon, giving a friend a call—whatever he wanted or needed to do that day. By the time he finished his chores or catching up with his phone calls, Skylar would be up and raring to go, and Ethan would forget about the computer entirely.

Can you guess what happened? After only four weeks or so, the pull of the computer every Monday at noon had weakened to the point where he was no longer masturbating and thereby sustaining the synapses and neural pathways that dragged him in that direction. He'd abandoned his tracks, which quickly became so overgrown and deteriorated that the temptations derailed, so to speak, before reaching him.

The fact is, your maleness and your human neuroplastic brain may have done you in when it came to your sexuality. But you are not a victim, and you are certainly not without hope. You simply must learn to effectively deal with your maleness if you want total victory over sexual sin. You have a decision to make.

7

Choosing True Manhood

You stand before an important battle. You've decided that the slavery of sexual sin isn't worth your love of sexual sin. You're committed to removing every hint of it. But how? Some of your male qualities loom as your own worst enemy.

If we got into sexual sin naturally—partly just by being male—then how do we get out? We can't eliminate our maleness, and we really don't want to. For instance, we want to look at our wives and desire them. They're beautiful to us, and we're sexually gratified when we gaze at them, often daydreaming about the night ahead and what bedtime will bring to both of us. In its proper place, maleness is wonderful.

Yet our maleness is a major root of sexual sin. So what do we do?

We must choose to be more than male. We must choose manhood.

From Fred: Maleness Versus Manhood

But what exactly is manhood? The best description I've read comes from author John Eldredge, who wrote the following in his classic book on maleness, *Wild at Heart:*

> There are three desires I find written so deeply into my heart I know now I can no longer disregard them without losing my soul. They are core to who and what I am and yearn to be. I gaze into boyhood, I search the pages of literature, I listen carefully to many, many men, and I am convinced these desires are universal, a clue into masculinity itself. They may be misplaced,

forgotten, or misdirected, but in the heart of every man is a desperate desire for a battle to fight, an adventure to live, and a beauty to rescue.[*]

I'll never forget the first time I read that last sentence. Eldredge said these words so simply, and yet what lay there on the page was *so* infinite and profound. I instantly recognized these same three desires throbbing in my *own* heart.

And the longer I thought about it, the more I saw that these were also the same three desires that energized my drive to sexual purity: *they are at the core of who I am and who I yearn to be.* The yearning burned, and declaring war provided me with everything a man's heart could desire:

- A huge battle to fight, whose end was uncertain
- A great adventure to live, grappling with the most heinous of enemies
- A life as a hero, coming through in the finest way I've ever found to protect my beauty

By becoming pure, I rescued my wife's dreams for marriage and motherhood. How heroic! I'd never felt more like a man, and it continues to this day.

When you choose manhood, you are choosing to be true to your created core. You are choosing to find and fight big battles for God, to live out great adventures in His kingdom, and to protect the beauty in your life, especially your wife and kids. That's what life for genuine men has always been about. Eldredge said that these three desires are universal, clues to masculinity itself, and while these desires may have been misplaced, forgotten, or misdirected in your life up until now, I know personally that taking on the battle for purity provides one strong way to restore order to your male core by freeing you to fight and crush the Enemy.

Before this battle, I'd had outstanding success as an athlete and a young businessman, but deep inside, I still doubted whether I truly belonged in the world of men. It was *this* purity battle and *this* adventure that established my manhood for good. I belong.

When our fathers admonished us to "be a man about it," they were encouraging us to rise to a standard of manhood they already understood. They wanted us

---

[*] John Eldredge, *Wild at Heart: Discovering the Secret of a Man's Soul* (Nashville: Thomas Nelson, 2001), 9.

to fulfill our potential, to rise above our natural tendencies to take the easy way out. When our fathers said, "Be a man," they were asking us to be like them, to fight, to live, to protect the beauty and the good.

In a similar way, our heavenly Father exhorts us higher, to be like Him: "The LORD is a warrior; the LORD is his name" (Exodus 15:3). While He knows His standard of purity doesn't come naturally to us, He calls us to rise above our natural tendencies to have impure eyes, fanciful minds, and wandering hearts. We are to be warriors by the power of His indwelling presence—to step into manhood, to fight fiercely, to live adventurously, and to protect heroically.

And that indwelling presence is enough in the battle. The apostle Peter tells us that this new life gives us everything we need as men to walk above our nature:

> His divine power has given us *everything we need* for a godly life through our knowledge of him who called us by his own glory and goodness. Through these he has given us his very great and precious promises, so that through them you may *participate in the divine nature, having escaped the corruption in the world* caused by evil desires. (2 Peter 1:3–4)

Before an important battle for the army he commanded, Joab said to the troops of Israel, "Be of good courage, and let us play the men for our people" (2 Samuel 10:12, KJV). In short, he was saying, "We know God's plan for us. Let's rise up as men and set our hearts and minds to get it done!"

It's time to play the man. Regarding sexual integrity, you've got the indwelling power, and soon you will have the knowledge that you need to win.

Rise up, O warrior! Choose manhood and get it done.

Jesus's Hands and Eyes

I understood better how manhood looks after reading a newsletter by author and speaker Dr. Gary Rosberg. In it, he told of seeing a pair of hands that reminded him of the hands of his father, who had gone on to heaven. Gary continued to reminisce about what his father's hands meant to him. Then he shifted his thoughts to the hands of Jesus, noting this simple truth: "They were hands that never touched a woman with dishonor."

As I read this line, sorrow tore at my soul. Oh, how I wished I could say that about my hands! I had degraded women with my hands, and I regretted the sin. As I thought about it further, though, I realized that since my first year of salvation, I hadn't touched a woman in dishonor. What a joy to contemplate!

I pondered Gary's words a little longer. Jesus's hands never touched a woman with dishonor, but He said that lusting with the eyes is the same as touching. Given that Jesus is sinless, I suddenly realized that He not only never *touched* a woman with dishonor, but He never even *looked* at a woman in dishonor, always having His eyes under control. Could I also say that?

I couldn't. Though saved and free to walk purely by His indwelling presence, I had still chosen to look at women in dishonor.

Oh, don't be so hard on yourself, one might say. *It's natural for a male to look. That's part of our nature.*

But you see, it is that exact mind-set that will keep you trapped in mere maleness rather than rising up into manhood. Sure, it may be natural for a *male* to look, but you are a *warrior,* called to crucify your lowest nature.

Let me illustrate how manhood looks in practice with a few stories I first shared in our workbook *Every Single Man's Battle.*

Several years ago, I slumped into the aisle seat on my flight to Dallas, where I would teach at a weekend men's retreat on sexual purity. As I rested my elbow on the armrest and laid my head on my hand, my eyes focused aimlessly as my fellow passengers filtered by. I was exhausted, and I hoped my seatmate would arrive quickly so that I could stand up one last time and then plop down to grab forty winks.

A young woman caught my eye with a faint smile and a nod toward her seat, which was next to mine. I stood up politely to let her squeeze in, and then I settled down to buckle up. About ten minutes after takeoff, I absentmindedly glanced out the window at the billowing clouds. As I did, I noticed this young woman had already laid her head back to sleep, and her low-cut top was offering a feast for my eyes. Was I tempted? Nah. I simply turned the other way. At this point in my life, a lingering peek down a woman's open blouse wasn't going to happen. Regarding the pretty young woman next to me, everything had already been settled in my mind years ago. My brain's train tracks for illicit glances were covered with an overgrowth of trees and brush, and the synaptic pathways were blocked from lack of use. Transformation is transformation, after all.

As I fell asleep in my aisle seat, I pondered what would have happened earlier in my life. My eyes would have roamed all over her, using her body for my selfish, sexual foreplay without her consent. *No, it would've been worse than that,* I mused. *I'd have been using her without her knowledge!*

Then suddenly it hit me. Peeking down her shirt as she slept would really be no different than, say, watching her through her window with a telescope as she undressed some evening. Using her here on the plane would have been just as premeditated, just as deceptive, and every bit as creepy as that.

I shivered. *Man, I never thought of it quite like that before—and to think I used to lust like that all the time!*

Some may wonder about my choice to do the right thing on the airplane. *So what? She wouldn't have known if you were looking at her!* That's irrelevant. I would have been using her for a sexual pop without her consent or even her knowledge. That's just plain degrading for any of us, as degrading as upskirting with your smartphone. Heroic men don't do that.

Besides, I'm also married. I'm not entitled to use her sexually in this way, whether or not she was aware of it. According to Jesus, that's a form of adultery, so end of discussion (see Matthew 5:27–28).

Before I move on, I want you to consider something else about this young woman. She is a daughter of the Most High God, and the Lord longs for her sexual purity and emotional protection. As His son, I am responsible to treat her with absolute purity, like a sister (see 1 Timothy 5:2). That's how genuine men live.

Years ago, when I was attending another church, the senior high youth pastor was fired for sexual misconduct with a vulnerable seventeen-year-old girl from the church. While my heart broke for this teen, his dismissal barely raised an eyebrow with me because I'd seen the red flags flying in his life for months.

The day after the firing, though, I *was* shattered by an incredible, indelible sight—something my heart begs to never see again as long as I live. My dear friend Randy, a local business owner and a close friend of the victim's family, stumbled shakily into my office to discuss the ugly matter, his face contorted with rage and torment nearly beyond recognition.

"Fred, how could he?" Randy murmured. "She was so young and vulnerable. She needed his protection, not this . . . How could this happen?" He then burst into heart-wrenching sobs.

Much later that morning, as his emotions finally ebbed, Randy told me something I'll never forget. "Fred, I have dozens of young women working for me in my stores, and do you know what I hear constantly from them? They tell me, 'Randy, I've never been around a man like you. I've never been able to trust a man in my life—not even my father, my brothers, my cousins—nobody. You're the only man I've ever felt safe to be around.'"

The tears came rolling again. "I can't tell you how much I cherish those words and the responsibility I carry. I fight with every fiber of my being to honor those girls who work for me. I'm sure some of them have been raped or molested at home, but now they've actually been able to see God in me, Fred. How could anyone violate such a trust, especially a youth pastor? I *have* to be honorable with these women in my care!"

My friend is "playing the man" well, isn't he? There would be no #MeToo movement today if all guys lived like Randy. Somewhere, sometime, he chose manhood, and he now lives out a great adventure every day protecting the women in his life instead of using them.

It's time to start honoring women with our eyes and with our minds. They're entitled to nothing less, and we're entitled to nothing more.

After all, we're men. This is what real men do. Sure, that girl sitting next to me on the plane fell asleep too soon to notice whether or not I'd lust or turn away from her in honor. But I'd chosen manhood years ago, and today I act the same way when no one is looking as I do when I'm sitting in the sanctuary of my home church. That is perhaps *the* key component of true manhood. Are you the same person regardless of where you are or who is watching?

In this arena, Jesus was definitely all man. Having never even *looked* on a woman with dishonor, He is clearly our role model.

Well, sure! you say. *He was God. It's unfair to expect me to live like Him!*

Maybe. But He was *fully man*! And if, because of His deity, Jesus's personal standard seems unattainable to you, let's look at another role model of manhood from Scripture in the area of sexual purity.

Just a Man

His name was Job, and in our minds this man is the essential human role model of sexual purity in Scripture. In the book of the Bible that tells his story, we see God bragging about Job to Satan:

> Have you considered my servant Job? There is no one on earth like him; he is blameless and upright, a man who fears God and shuns evil. (Job 1:8)

Was God proud of Job? You bet! He applauded His servant's faithfulness in words of highest praise. And if you walked in purity, blameless and upright, He would speak just as proudly of you. Joy would abound in His heart. You already have the freedom and authority to walk purely.

But such a passage from Scripture may actually discourage you when you compare Job's example with your own life. So let's find out more about how Job did it.

In Job 31:1, we see Job making this startling revelation: "I made a covenant with my eyes not to look lustfully at a young woman."

A covenant with his eyes! You mean he made a promise with his eyes to not gaze upon a young woman? It's not possible! It can't be true!

Yet Job was totally successful; otherwise, he wouldn't have made this promise:

> If my heart has been enticed by a woman,
> or if I have lurked at my neighbor's door,
> then may my wife grind another man's grain,
> and may other men sleep with her. (verses 9–10)

Job had engaged the big battle and lived out the great adventure. He knew he had lived right, and he knew his eyes and mind were pure. He swore to it upon his wife and marriage before God and man.

Let's go back to the beginning of the story and read the opening verse of the book of Job:

> In the land of Uz there lived *a man* whose name was Job. This *man* was blameless and upright; he feared God and shunned evil.

Did you catch it? Job was just a man, like you and me! As you realize that, these precious words should gloriously flood your soul: *If he can do it, so can I.* God wants you to know that if you step into manhood, you, too, can rise above sexual impurity.

From Fred: Making My Covenant

When I first gave serious consideration to Job's example, I meditated upon his words for days on end. Job and I were different in only one way: our actions. God called him "blameless." I wasn't yet blameless, but I was a man, just as Job was, so there was hope.

After a few days, my mind turned to the word *covenant*—an agreement between God and a person. What exactly was I to do when I made a covenant? I could say the words to make a promise, but I was uncertain whether I could keep my word.

And my eyes? Could I really expect my eyes to keep their end of the bargain? Eyes can't think or talk! How do they keep a promise?

Day after day, my mind returned to this covenant concept, trying to picture it, all the while remaining in my sin. Yet something was stirring deep in my soul.

I remember the moment—the exact spot on Merle Hay Road in Des Moines—when it all broke loose. I'd just failed God with my eyes for the thirty-millionth time by lusting over a jogger. My heart churned in guilt, pain, and sorrow. I suddenly gripped the wheel, and through clenched teeth I yelled out, "That's it! I'm through with this! I'm making a covenant with my eyes. I don't care what it takes, and I don't care if I die trying. It stops here. It stops here!"

I made that covenant and built it brick by brick. Later, Steve and I will show you the blueprint for building that brick wall, but for now, study the simple nature of my breakthrough:

- I made a clear decision.
- I decided once and for all to make a change.

I can't describe how much I meant it. A flood of frustration from years of failure poured from my heart. I'd just had it! I wasn't fully convinced I could trust myself even then, but I'd finally and truly engaged the battle. Through my covenant with my eyes, all my mental and spiritual resources were now leveled upon a single target: my impurity.

In short, I had also chosen manhood. I'd taken on the big battle to rise above my natural male tendencies, and I'd embarked on a great adventure to put the Enemy under my feet.

Part III

Choosing Victory

8

The Time to Decide

We came across a newspaper story about a World War II vet named B. J. "Bernie" Baker who was told he was dying of bone cancer. Given only two years to live, he told the doctors to fight the disease with everything possible. "Give me the treatments," he said. "I'll keep living my life." Meanwhile, he and his wife found time for a motor-home drive to Alaska, a fishing excursion to Costa Rica, and several trips to Florida.

Nine years after the diagnosis, he was struggling with shortage of breath and loss of strength but said, "I'm going to keep fighting. Might as well."

Those words were not said in resignation. They were the words of a fighter, a real man, a man who had faced bombs and machine-gun fire in the South Pacific before returning to America and eventually starting Baker Mechanical with two pipe wrenches and a $125 pickup truck. (It would become one of the largest companies of its kind in America.) The cancer hit him hard, but he had no plans for surrender.

Might as well keep fighting. What was B. J.'s alternative?

To quit and die.

What about you in your battle with impure eyes and mind? What's your alternative to fighting?

To stay ensnared and die spiritually.

When you talk to courageous men from B. J.'s generation, World War II veterans who embody the title of Tom Brokaw's book *The Greatest Generation*, they say they simply had a job to do. When the landing-craft ramps fell open, those men swallowed hard and said, "It's time." Time to fight.

In your struggle with sexual impurity, isn't it time? Sure, fighting back will be hard. It was for us. When we began our fight, we fully expected to take a beating at first, and we did. Our sin had humbled us. But we wanted victory over that sin and the respect of our God.

Your life and home are under a withering barrage of machine-gun sexuality that rakes the landscape mercilessly. Right now you're in a landing craft, inching closer to shore and a showdown. God has given you the weapons and trained you for battle.

You can't stay in the landing craft forever. Sooner or later, the ramp will drop, and then it will be your time to run bravely into the teeth of battle. God will run *with* you, but He won't run *for* you.

It's time to plunge ahead and go like a man.

From Fred: Winning When the Battle Is Hottest

If you remember my story, I dumped the pornography before my wedding day, but since I hadn't entirely stopped yielding to our sexual culture's negative influence upon me, I remained ensnared. Eventually, I became so tired of the battle that I just wanted it to go away.

I was angry too. I was sick of sinning, sick of Satan, and sick of me. I didn't want to wait anymore. Like the people of Israel, I came to loathe myself (see Ezekiel 6:9). I wanted to win right away and to win decisively, not somewhere down the road where aging might bring victory through the back door. I wanted to win when the battle was hottest.

You should too. If you don't win now, you'll never know whether you're a man of God who's truly after His purposes.

Going to War, Going to Win

Sexual sin isn't just a game out there, just one more form of scintillating entertainment. It warps the pathways to your brain's pleasure centers. It literally changes your sexual tastes, and it will lock you up spiritually and throw away the key. If you're going to engage the battle, know this: you've got to fight for keeps. There will be no victory in this area of your life until you choose manhood and choose victory with all your might.

Leading up to a decisive choice for sexual purity, you must make some hard choices and answer some hard questions:

- How long do you intend to stay ensnared?
- How long must your family wait?
- How long before you can look God in the eye again?

Brenda asked me one of those hard questions many years ago, and I can still feel the impact as if it were yesterday. Although the topic that afternoon focused on something other than sexual sin, the story behind it illustrates the hard decisions necessary to escape sexual bondage.

When I reached age thirty-five, the fact that my dad had never accepted me as a man rocked me deeply, right out of the blue. Inner pain seeped out and affected my relationship with my wife and kids. I was harsh in my tone, harsh in my words. Harsh, harsh, harsh.

Again and again, Brenda tried to explain away my behavior to the kids, but after a full year of mounting frustration, one day she erupted, "All right, then! Fine. Just tell all of us how long you plan to stay like this so we can prepare for it!" Then she stormed out of the room and slammed the door.

I sat there speechless for some time. Sure, her rage shocked me, but her point shocked me most. Just exactly how long *was* I going to stay like this? Ten years? Why ten? Why not five? And if I could simply decide to change at the end of five years, why not after one? And if after one, why not now?

After her single stiletto question to my heart, I knew it was time to mobilize. Starting immediately, I found a counselor. Shortly after that, I attended a Promise Keepers conference in Colorado. That first night, God revealed an aspect of His unconditional love for me that I'd never understood before. Sitting that evening in the bleachers at the University of Colorado's Folsom Field, the pain from years of my dad's verbal abuse dispersed in mere moments.

My family deserved more than what I'd been delivering. After all, I was a man.

Men fight big battles, live great adventures, and defend the beauty in their lives. I had to act decisively in the face of Brenda's challenge.

More Questions

In the same way, you're at your own point of decision in the arena of sexual purity. Your family deserves more than you're delivering in this regard, and they're awaiting your response. It's time you embark on your own great adventure and fight a big battle to defend your family.

But unlike it was with Brenda, your own wife may not even be aware of your problem with sexual impurity, so she can't ask you the hard questions. If that's the case, we'll ask those questions for her:

- How long are you going to stay sexually impure?
- How long will you rob your wife sexually?
- How long will you stunt the growth of oneness with your wife, a oneness you promised her years ago before many witnesses in a wedding ceremony?

God's view is clear here. You need to face those questions and make a decision. Yet you're hesitating. We understand. We hesitated for years ourselves. You're thinking, *Wait a minute. I'm not ready.* Or perhaps this thought is center stage: *I'd quit today, but it just isn't that easy!*

Fine. We'll agree that choosing to stop sinning doesn't seem very simple. Once you're ensnared, everything looks complex. But listen to the following words spoken in a sermon by the late evangelist Steve Hill, who was addressing his personal escape from addiction to drugs and alcohol, as well as from sexual sin:

> There's no temptation that is uncommon to man. God will send you a way of escape, but you've got to be willing to take that way of escape, friend. . . .
>
> I was an alcoholic to the max. I would drink whiskey, straight whiskey, every day. And I was a junkie. Cocaine up my nose, in my arm . . . I did it all, friend. And God never delivered me from the desire and the love of drugs. He

never did. What happened is that I decided to never touch the stuff or drink booze again. . . .

Those of you that are into pornography may be asking God to take away your lustful desires. You are a man with hormones. You feel things. You have since you were a teenager, and you will until the day you die! You are attracted to the opposite sex.

I'm not saying that God cannot take the desire from you. He can! He's just never done it in my life or the tens of thousands of people I've worked with over the years. That includes pornographers. Ninety-nine percent of them had to make a decision. They had to make a decision to not walk by magazine racks of adult magazines and to stay faithful to their wives and their family.

We agree. Everything starts with a decision. It's time to make one.

How long will you dally? Will you wait ten years and then choose to stop? If not ten years, what about five years? One year?

Why not now?

From Fred: This Is Your Moment

As you deliberate, consider the example of Eleazar, one of King David's "three mighty warriors" (2 Samuel 23:9), in this brief record of a tough battle against the Philistines:

The Israelites retreated, but Eleazar stood his ground and struck down the Philistines till his hand grew tired and froze to the sword. The Lord brought about a great victory that day. (verses 9–10)

Eleazar refused to be ensnared any longer. Everyone else ran from the enemy, but he put his foot down and said, "I'm not running. I will fight until I drop dead or until I drop to the field in victorious exhaustion. This is my moment, live or die."

Have you had it with the running? Is this your moment?

Author and pastor Jack Hayford once spoke of his moment. Sitting in his car after a banking transaction with a lovely bank teller, he said to himself, *I'm either going to have to purify my mind and consecrate myself unto God, or I'm going to have to masturbate right here.* Pastor Jack said this in front of fifty thousand men at the same Promise Keepers conference I spoke of earlier. When was the last time you could have heard a pin drop in a completely filled football stadium?

Like Eleazar, Jack Hayford stood his ground, snarling, "I've had it with this running. It stops here!" And the Lord brought about a great victory that day.

How about you? How long will you allow the Philistines to chase you? Are you motivated instead to fight? This could be *your* moment.

Motivated to Win

Let me (Fred) share one last story of a guy who once became very motivated to change. Several weeks prior to his planned wedding, he heard me give a talk on sexual purity. My words weighed heavily on his heart because he was having a problem with sexy R-rated movies and the masturbation that sometimes followed. He had been planning to marry Heather with his secret safely tucked away, but now he decided to tell her the truth.

Heather recalls her reaction to Barry's confession: "I was shocked and numb when we talked in the car that night. I just stared straight ahead, no feelings at all.

"After dropping him off, I cried and cried, refusing to talk to him for days. When I did agree to see him, he commented to me that I looked pretty. Rage stormed through me as I realized that his definition of *pretty* was formed by the filthy women he'd been watching in those movies. I got so mad and repulsed by him that I threw the engagement ring in his face and told him to get out of my sight. I felt sick and dirty."

As you can see, this topic is an emotional one. Women take it personally when they find out what men are doing in secret.

Heather asked Brenda and me to meet with her, which we did. After much prayer and counseling, Heather gave Barry a deadline of one week to dump the sin.

Then I met with Barry. "Can you help me?" he asked. "I'm absolutely hooked on sensual movies. I expected Heather to understand, but she was horrified and called me a pervert. Fred, I'm desperate! The wedding invitations have already been sent out, but if I don't get this stopped, I'll have to somehow explain all this to my mother-in-law! You've got to help me!"

Do you suppose Barry was motivated? He surely was. Rarely have I met with someone who wanted to win a war more quickly. It was his moment, and he defeated that huge adversary. He became a man of sexual integrity practically overnight, and today he and Heather have a wonderful marriage.

You can win the war as well—and start winning it now.

God Is Waiting

As we said earlier, you already have everything you need inside to win this battle (see 2 Peter 1:3–4), just like Barry and every other Christian guy. In the millisecond it takes to make that choice, the Holy Spirit will start guiding you and walking through the struggle with you.

After all, it's God's will for you to have sexual purity, though you may not think so since this hasn't been your constant experience. But read this scripture:

> It is God's will that you should be sanctified: that you should avoid sexual immorality; that each of you should learn to control your own body in a way that is holy and honorable. (1 Thessalonians 4:3–4)

God is waiting for you. But He is not waiting by the altar at church, hoping you'll drop by for the umpteenth time to cry for a while. He is already out on the battlefield, glancing at His watch, waiting for you to arrive and rise up and engage in the battle. You have the spiritual power through the Lord to overcome every level of sexual immorality, but if you don't stand up and utilize that power, you'll never break free of the habit.

You see, sexual impurity isn't like a tumor growing out of control inside you. You treat it that way when your prayers focus on some dramatic spiritual intervention, like deliverance, as you plead for someone to come remove it. Actually, sexual impurity is a series of bad decisions on your part—sometimes as a result of immature character—and deliverance won't deliver you into instant maturity. Character work needs to be done so that the warped synaptic pathways in your brain can die, as grace "teaches us to say 'No' to ungodliness and worldly passions, and to live self-controlled, upright and godly lives in this present age" (Titus 2:12).

Remember this: holiness is not some nebulous, mystical thing. You needn't wait around for some holy cloud to form around you. From the perspective of daily practice, it's simply a series of right choices. You'll be holy when you choose not to sin.

By God's grace, you're already free from the power of sexual immorality. But you are not yet free from the *habit* of sexual immorality until you choose to be— until you say, "That's enough! I'm choosing to live purely!"

It's Time

So then, God is waiting to bless you.

Your wife needs you to step up.

Your kids need you to break the generational sin.

Do you agree it's time?

Good. Let's put together a battle plan. The landing-craft ramps are falling open, and it's time to hit the beach.

9

Your Battle Plan 1:
Winning Is the Objective

B efore we started winning our own battles for purity, we had a number of false starts—partly because we hadn't really made an unshakable decision. We sort of wanted purity and sort of didn't. Furthermore, we didn't understand the Enemy or how to approach this battlefield. The whole business of sexual integrity was mysterious.

Let's say you're in the landing craft, ready to attack your sexual sin. You've made your decision. You've decided to follow your leaders as you storm the beach. The landing-craft ramp falls open. With a shout, you step courageously into the fray. But, unknown to you, the deceptive ocean currents have flushed a deep hole on the ocean floor right in front of the landing craft. You have no idea what's happened, but you're suddenly in water over your head and the weight of your pack is sending you to the bottom. You're drowning.

Your battle is over before you even take a second step.

Satan's greatest weapon against you is just such deception. He knows Jesus has already purchased your freedom. He also knows that once you see the simplicity of this battle, you'll win in short order, so he deceives and confuses. He whispers, tricking you into thinking you're a helpless victim, someone who'll need years of group therapy. *What's the point of trying, pal?*

He laughs at you and loves telling you that looking and lusting is just part of being a guy. *There's nothing you can do about it, so quit fighting it, dude. God wouldn't have made women this beautiful if He didn't want you to enjoy them this way.*

He soon has you believing that the brain studies are exaggerated and you don't really even have a problem. *There's nothing to all that. You don't have to live any differently from the guys at work.* Such deception is only one of the ways that Satan tries to beat you.

Your Objective in This War

Your goal is sexual purity. Here's a good working definition of it, good because of its simplicity: *you are sexually pure when you're getting no sexual gratification from anyone or anything but your wife.*

In other words, victory means stopping the sexual gratification that comes into you from outside marriage. But how do you stop it?

Well, you first need to ask where it comes from. The answer is that you're able to draw outside sexual gratification from only two places: the eyes and the mind. Therefore, to be successful in the battle, you must set up a sexual-defense perimeter to blockade the shipping lanes of the eyes and mind. Beyond that, you must also make sure you have healthy, positive affections and attitudes in your relationship with your wife. In other words, you want your heart to be right and to become one with hers.

That means your objective in the war against lust is to build a three-layered defense perimeter into your life:

1. With your eyes
2. In your mind
3. In your heart

Think of the first perimeter (your eyes) as your outermost defense, a wall with Keep Out signs around it. It defends your eyes by covenant (as Job did: "I made a covenant with my eyes not to look lustfully at a young woman," Job 31:1), and you do that by training your eyes to bounce away from objects of lust. Your eyes must bounce away from the sensual, something they aren't currently doing.

With the second perimeter (your mind), you don't so much block out the objects of lust, but rather you evaluate and capture them. A key verse to support you here is 2 Corinthians 10:5: "We take captive every thought to make it obedient to Christ." You must train your mind to intercept thoughts.

Your third objective is to build your innermost defense perimeter—in your heart. This perimeter is built by strengthening your affections for your wife and your commitment to the promises and debts you owe her. Your marriage can die from within if you neglect your promise to love, honor, and cherish your wife. (And this applies even if you're single: you want to honor and cherish every date, just as you hope every guy is honoring and cherishing your future wife when he goes out with her.)

We've purposely focused on defense because most men have never been taught how to defend the vulnerabilities of their male makeup. That's what you most need from us, and since this three-layered defense plan is crucial to your victory, we'll spend the rest of this book helping you set it up.

But remember that, in this rugged battle, your offense and defense must always take the field together. Praying for the supernatural power of the Holy Spirit to empower you is the best offensive move you can make, so don't sideline your offense as you build up your defense. Never forget that prayer isn't just for warm-ups or to prepare for a battle. It's in prayer that the battle can be won or lost.

For example, when Jesus was praying in the Garden of Gethsemane, His prayer time *was* the battle, and it was so intense that He sweat drops of blood. When He prayed that, if possible, God would take away all the pain He was about to endure, He was already winning. By the time He was finished praying, Satan was on the run because the mind and heart of Christ were set to do whatever the Father had in store for Him. Once that victory had been won in prayer in the garden, there was no question what would happen on Jesus's way to the Cross. So again, never sideline your offense, even as you begin building your defenses. Get away with God to your own garden and engage this battle in prayer.

So there's your battle plan. That's it. Nothing more, nothing less. In prayerfully setting up these three defense perimeters, you're simultaneously choosing not to sin. You'll have freedom from sexual impurity as soon as these defense perimeters are in place. Sexually speaking, your outer life will match the inner life God created in you. You'll finally be exactly who people think you are and exactly who you say you are.

Because of your long struggle with sexual impurity, this attack plan may seem too simple to be effective. But as you study the attributes of your enemy, you'll realize that simplicity is more than sufficient.

Before we move on to how to build the three defense perimeters, let's remove some of the mystery surrounding sexual sin and gain a better understanding of the Enemy so that you might not be deceived on the battlefield.

Impurity Is a Habit

Far too often, men see themselves as a victim of their genetics: *I'm male, so it's a given. I'm going to have impure eyes and an impure mind.* But we can't blame our roving eyes on genetics, even though our Y chromosome definitely makes us more visually oriented than women. In spite of that, our genetics do not absolve us from all responsibility.

The simple truth? Impurity is a habit. It lives like a habit. When some hot-looking babe walks in, your eyes have the bad habit of bouncing toward her and then sliding up and down. When some glistening jogger runs past you, your eyes habitually run away with her. When the *Sports Illustrated* swimsuit issue arrives every February, out of habit you fantasize over the curves and crevices, fondling every arresting image in sexual foreplay with your eyes.

The fact that impurity is merely a habit comes as a surprise to many men. It's like discovering that the big bully has a glass chin and that you don't have to cower anymore.

If impurity were genetic or some victimizing spell, you'd be helpless. But since impurity is a habit, it can be changed. You have hope because if it lives like a habit, it can die like a habit. For Fred, it took about six weeks to change his eye habits, but admittedly, that is on the short end of normal. Caroline Leaf's studies on the neuroplasticity of habit change suggests a slightly longer time frame may be necessary for others. She aptly warns, "As they say, Rome wasn't built in a day. It takes time to change, so give yourself a break if you do make a mistake or fail! . . . It takes a minimum of 63 days to change an automated habit—when it comes to the mind, there really are no quick fixes and most people give up on day 4, so be patient!"[*]

Whether it takes forty-two days or sixty-three days for you is immaterial. What matters is that impurity is merely a habit. This is great news since habit breaking is familiar ground, hardly mysterious. We've all dealt with bad habits. What do you do with them? You simply replace them with new and better ones. That's it. If you can practice this new habit with great focus for six to nine weeks, soon the old habit will seem unnatural.

The latest science backs up our position that impurity lives like a habit. Brian Anderson is a cognitive neuroscientist with a specialty in habit formation. His research shows that visual stimuli linked to a reward—think dopamine—are harder to ignore when encountered again. In other words, when your brain identifies evidence of a gratifying sensual stimulus in the environment around you, it will pay more attention and also block out other stimuli.[†]

Your brain is wired to establish these patterns, like continually looking lustfully at the women around you. When you tie such habits to visual pleasure, they can be troublesome and tough to break. In short, your sexual visual nature lends itself to a strong and quick attention bias, and because of the reward neurotransmitter involved, your brain is going to learn that association promptly and wire it in.

Clearly, then, sexual impurity is not a sickness or imbalance for most men. Our eyes simply love the sexual, and our bad habits arise from our maleness and this attention bias. We have the bad habit of seeking cheap thrills from any dark corner we stumble into. We've habitually chosen the wrong way, and now we must habitually choose the right way instead.

Don't misunderstand—we're not saying your habits have no relationship to your emotions or circumstances. Glen told us, "My sexual sin became much worse when I was under a deadline at work and especially whenever my wife and I fought or I felt unloved and unappreciated. It seemed at those times that I was compelled to sin sexually and couldn't say no. Honestly, I didn't think that would ever change simply

---

[*] Dr. Caroline Leaf, "Why We Keep Making the Same Mistakes + Tips to Break Bad Habits," *Dr. Leaf's Blog,* May 9, 2019, https://drleaf.com/blog/why-we-keep-making-the-same-mistakes-tips-to-break-bad-habits.

[†] Belinda Luscombe, "Porn and the Threat to Virility," *Time,* March 31, 2016, http://time.com/magazine /us/4277492/april-11th-2016-vol-187-no-13-u-s.

by changing the habits of my eyes. But guess what? Once I got my eyes under control, these same deadlines and fights no longer compelled me sexually. My impurity just seemed to wither away on its own."

In Glen's case, the sexual impurity was simply one way he dealt with these emotions and stressful circumstances. In short, he ran to impurity as an escape. But once he removed the sexual impurity, he began processing these things in other ways, nonsexually.

Impurity Works like a Habit

Impurity not only *lives* like a habit but also *works* like a habit. The same is true for purity: it works like a habit.

What do we mean?

Once we set a habit in concrete, we can forget about it. The habit will take care of business with little conscious thought, enabling us to focus our attention on other things. For example, we all have a habitual way of getting up in the morning. Many of us slowly climb out of bed, brush our teeth, take a shower, get dressed, and eat Wheaties with the kids at 7:10 a.m. We don't even have to think about it. We could do our morning routine in our sleep, and we usually do!

While sexual impurity works like a *bad* habit, sexual purity works like a *good* habit, as simply and consistently as getting up and going off to work in the morning. It can be effortless.

This should be encouraging to you. As you enter the fight against impurity, the exhausting battle might have you saying to yourself, *I can't work this hard at purity the rest of my life.* Well, you don't have to. If you can just hang in there a little longer, the good habit of purity will get a foothold and will then fight for you naturally, requiring much less conscious effort over time.

Currently, your impure habits claw and clutch; you sin without even thinking. For instance, your eyes bounce to any short skirt that moseys by. Without thinking, your bad habits kick in. But once the habit of purity is in place, when a woman's dress flies up on a windy day, you'll look away instantly and automatically without even thinking. If you wanted to peek, you'd have to force your eyes to do so.

From Fred: Forcing a Look

Hard to imagine? Then consider this little story. After having trained my eyes to look away, I was sunbathing with Brenda on a Florida beach. Brenda called my attention to a bikini-clad woman approaching us. "Fred, look! You won't believe this!"

Initially I couldn't turn to look. The good habits had become so strong that I had to force my eyes to do so.

"She's way too old to wear that!" Brenda said about the seventy-something woman. I'm not sure what surprised me more at the time: having to force my eyes to look at a woman in a bikini or seeing someone that old wearing something that skimpy!

Impurity Fights like an Addiction

Impurity of the eyes and mind lives and works like a habit, but it also *fights* like an addiction. Many habits are addictive. Smokers get the urge to smoke. Drug users "get a jones." Alcoholics get the shakes.

For overcoming some addictions, the addictive source can be gradually reduced. For others, the best method is cold turkey. What works best with sexual impurity? Cold turkey. You cannot just taper down. We tried. It didn't work because we found our minds and eyes were too tricky and deceitful. With tapering, whatever impurity you *do* allow seems to multiply in its impact, and the habit won't break. Remember how your warped synaptic pathways live or die on a use-it-or-lose-it basis? With tapering, you're still using and maintaining the very pathways you want to kill. That doesn't advance the ball down the field.

Besides, tapering down also brings with it the possibility of sexual binges that might go on for days. Binges crush your spirit. "I used to try to stop my sexual sin without really understanding what I was fighting," said Cliff. "I might grit my teeth and do well for a while, but then suddenly, maybe because I hadn't had sex in a while or because of some lustful thoughts that just got carried away, I would masturbate. Then I would say to myself, *Well, since I failed, I might as well fail big.* I would masturbate two, three times a day for the next week or two before I could get back the strength to fight again. I can't tell you how many times I've binged like this."

Cold turkey it must be. But how? By totally starving your eyes of all things sensual besides your wife. We'll teach you how to starve your eyes later in part 4, but for now, know that you can expect an inner "urge to fail" at times. You're accustomed to satisfying a portion of your sexual hunger through your eyes anytime and anywhere you please. Your body will fight to maintain this freedom and these highs. As you advance in purity, the part of your sexual hunger that was once fed by your eyes will remain unfed. That demanding hunger doesn't just disappear, but it will run to the only available pantry left to you: your wife. In chapter 11, you'll see more about how this works out to satisfy both of you.

Spiritual Possession and Oppression

We touched earlier on Satan's part in our battle against impurity, but now let's focus on whether sexual impurity represents some form of demon possession.

Our enemy is a liar, no question. We've mentioned his deceiving tactics already. But in truth, we believe that most of us give far too much credit to the Enemy when it comes to sexual sin. You aren't possessed by the devil when impurity runs rampant in your life, and you don't need anything like an exorcism. Granted, sometimes you'd swear an evil gremlin is inside you, yanking you about and driving you to sin, but these feelings are merely the compulsions of your bad habits and your brain's craving for its hit of drugs.

From Fred: The Enemy or Your Frenemy Brain?

I used to travel a lot for my business. I hated hotel rooms because as soon as I slid my key into the slot and walked in, it seemed that about seventy demons rushed over me, and the horrible, yanking, choking temptations would set in. I felt so overmatched, one mere mortal against seventy immortals, and so it was way too easy to give in to sexual temptations.

Today, I can go into any hotel room in perfect peace. I haven't felt a temptation there for years. Where'd the demons go? The answer is easy: they were never there. Those "temptations" were nothing more than the subconscious yanking on my own synaptic pathways, crabbing, *What, we're in a hotel room? Then where's my hit of drugs?* Because these demands were subconscious and outside my will, I thought they were coming from outside me. But they weren't.

What you often think of as a "gremlin moment" is nothing more than your addicted brain responding to its present circumstances, demanding what it normally gets when you're in a hotel, in your shower at home, or in a particular bathroom stall in the corner of the student union.

But now, since I never give my eyes or brain a sensual thing in any hotel room at any time, the use-it-or-lose-it principle has kicked in. Those old, addictive synaptic pathways that once seemed demonic and that used to drag me into sin are dead.

While there's no spiritual possession involved, there could be an element of spiritual oppression. You be the judge in my case:

Near my six-week mark of going cold turkey, I had a very sensual and violent dream. I was tempted sexually in an extremely enticing manner, and yet, for the first time in a dream, I actually said, "No, I won't." (You'll know you're nearing victory when, even in the freedom of your dream state, your subconscious mind still chooses purity.)

Three times this gorgeous, demonic woman sneered, "You *will* make love to me." Three times, I snarled in return, "No, I won't." With that, she seized my throat and wrenched me onto the bed in violent hand-to-hand combat, and I cried out, "In the name of Jesus, I will defeat you!"

As I said the words "In the name of Jesus," the battle turned in my favor. But when I said the words "I will defeat you," the battle turned violently against me since I had no power of my own. In desperation, I cried out every name of Jesus I could think of: "Prince of Peace, Lord of lords, King of kings, Beautiful Savior . . ."

Suddenly, I awoke with a start, shouting praises to God at the top of my lungs. It was a Sunday morning.

Several hours later in church, I worshipped freely all service long for the first time. Praises continued to bubble up out of my heart the rest of the day, that night, and into the next day. For someone who had felt such distance from God for so long and hadn't been able to connect with Him effectively in worship, the feeling was glorious.

The explanation? I'm convinced a spiritual oppression in my life was crushed that night when I rejected the Enemy's claim on my sexuality. Obviously, I can't be dogmatic about this because it was a dream, after all, and because I've never been one to look for Satan behind every rock. All I know for certain is that before that night, I'd never been able to worship freely. After that night, worship flowed easily from my heart like a river of living water, and it continues to this day.

Defeating Satan's Lies

Whether or not your battle involves spiritual *oppression*, you will always face spiritual *opposition*. The Enemy is constantly near your ear. He doesn't want you to win this fight, and he knows the lies that so often break men's confidence and their will to win. Expect to hear lies and plenty of them.

What we've told you is the truth. There is peace and tranquility for you on the other side of this war. There is immeasurable spiritual gain. The Deceiver will tell you that Steve Arterburn and Fred Stoeker are crazy and that you'll soon be as crazy as both of them combined if you follow their instructions.

To help you recognize Satan's lies when you hear them, here's a list of some of them. (After each lie, we'll state the actual truth.)

Satan: "You're the only one dealing with this problem. If anyone ever finds out, you'll be the laughingstock of the church!"

The truth: Most men deal with this problem, so no one will laugh. If anything, they'll applaud your courage.

Satan: "You failed again. You'll never be able to train your eyes. It's impossible."

The truth: It isn't impossible. Job trained his eyes, didn't he? He was a man just like you. You've got this.

Satan: "You're being so legalistic! The law is dead and brings only death."

The truth: God still has standards of behavior for us, and you're responsible to live purely by His standards. Life flows from obedience.

Satan: "Oh, c'mon! Don't be such a moron. This 'habit-changing' plan will never work."

The truth: The plan will work because, for most men, the problem of sexual impurity is linked significantly to bad choices evolving into bad habits, which are eventually rooted into synaptic pathways maintained by dopamine rewards. Stop using the pathways, and the pathways disappear. It'll work.

Satan: "Why fight this costly battle when the costs of your impurity are so minimal?"

The truth: You can't always see them immediately, but the costs of your sin are greater than you think, including the compromise of your spiritual protection over your home and the passing on of the example of your own slack sexual habits with your eyes and your porn to your children.

Satan: "Why live in this high state of alert for the rest of your life? Give up now, and I'll leave you alone."

The truth: Satan just might keep his word and leave you alone, but even if he did, the laws of reaping and sowing would still exact their payment from you. You cannot avoid the costs of sexual impurity. You might as well fight.

Satan: "You'll be awkward in business situations now, especially with women. You won't fit in, and you'll lose business."

The truth: No, you won't be awkward in business situations. Without that low-grade sexual fever you've always felt around women, you'll be more at ease with them than ever.

Masturbation: A Symptom, Not the Root

If your sexual impurity includes masturbation, as it does for many men, then further discussion is necessary. Let's tackle this issue head on.

Let us say it clearly: masturbation is mostly a symptom of uncontrolled eyes and free-racing thoughts that launch your sex drive into hyperdrive. When you create the new habits of bouncing your eyes and taking thoughts captive, masturbation will largely cease. Until then, it won't. There's no sense in targeting masturbation itself because you won't be attacking the real source of the problem. Target the eyes and mind instead.

Scripture is silent on the topic of masturbation. Some make a case that isolated instances of masturbation to relieve sexual tension are okay, especially if you're focusing on your wife, not some supermodel, during periods of separation or illness.

We disagree.

There can be no question that wanton masturbation in marriage, tied to pornography or whatever gets the guy's motor running, is always out of line. First of all, the act puts a distance between you and God. If you desire holiness, you must stop masturbating. Second, it puts a distance between you and your wife in bed. If you desire tight sexual intimacy with her, you must stop masturbating.

If you want freedom from masturbation, you must put the ax to the roots. What are the roots? That you're stopping short of God's standard, accepting (through your eyes and your mind) more than a hint of immorality in your life.

Masturbation and Emotional Pain

A moment ago, we said, "When you create the new habits of bouncing your eyes and taking thoughts captive, masturbation will largely cease." The reason we say "largely" is because some masturbation may continue due to a second root beneath it.

Most of us get involved with masturbation early in our lives, and along the way we notice how the brain chemistry impacts us. We don't consciously see it, and we generally don't put two and two together, but over time we recognize that the chemistry of that orgasm medicates our pain. Masturbation becomes like an easily obtained feel-good drug. When we're down, when we are stressed, when our girlfriends have fought with us, we tend to run to porn and masturbation.

When you think of how an orgasm feels to a man, it makes sense that it works that way. At the point of climax, there is a feeling of control and dominance. Along with it, there is a feeling of completion and a fleeting sense of connection with another human soul. Because of the orgasm, masturbation can feel like intimacy to us, if only for a moment, and it can feel like we've reestablished control in our lives and circumstances—again, for only a moment. But to a lonely, hurting, and disconnected guy, the draw can be quite compelling.

Masturbation is the path of least resistance—a pretend lover, a pornographic lover with a permanent smile. A lover who never says no, one who never rejects. One who never abandons and is always discreet. One who supports the man's ego in the midst of his self-doubt, who forever says, "Everything will be okay," no matter how high the pressure goes. This path is a chosen path, a path made available by the impure eyes stoking the sexual fever, providing an unending pool of lovers from which to draw.

The reason rejection and masturbation coexist so often is because of our maleness and our easy ability to draw true sexual gratification through our eyes. The male eyes give us the means to sin broadly and at will. Then, because men get their intimacy from the acts just prior to and during intercourse, masturbation brings a real sense of intimacy and acceptance. This sense of intimacy, often called false intimacy, temporarily salves the hurt and rejection. False intimacy is attained easily and without risk, far more easily than at some bar or whorehouse. In fact, it's attained more easily than with a wife, who might say no when you are desiring—or hurting—the most. That's why men choose to masturbate so often.

What if the means to sin are taken away by training the eyes? Masturbation is no longer the path of least resistance. Hopefully the man will finally deal with the rejection itself. But the masturbation? It goes away. Men don't *have* to masturbate because they've been traumatized emotionally. They're *choosing it* as just one more means, one more drug of forgetfulness, to deal with their pain.

From Fred: Fighting On for Victory

So, you may still have a bit of a fight going on even after you do get your eyes under control. I got mine under control by the end of six weeks, and I assumed the battle was over. Those were wonderful days, an awesome time of many glorious victories, and my relationship with God blossomed in wonderful ways in the weeks and months that followed. Compared to the first six weeks of heavy warfare, the rest of the battle seemed like mop-up duty or a downhill march.

But I still had to deal with some very stiff pockets of resistance when it came to my masturbation habit. While my eyes were finally under control, for instance, my mind was still hopelessly out of control with fantasies for a time, and while my masturbation habit had been weakened severely by that covenant with my eyes, it would still be about three more years before I masturbated for the last time—even though I was married and having all the sex I wanted.

Surprised? Don't be. Masturbation, while obviously sexual in nature, can certainly have nonsexual roots, like the ones I mentioned above. Sure, there are sexual triggers to masturbation, such as watching a Netflix series littered with sexual scenes and themes, but there are also emotional triggers, like the stress of work and even old wounds from our fathers.

In my estimation, the emotional triggers to masturbate can be as strong as the sexual triggers, and your masturbation habit may actually be more of an emotional addiction than a sexual one. That's why guys who cut the porn and the eye candy may still find themselves addicted to masturbation.

The important point is that my defeats during this mop-up time were absolutely critical to my eventual victory. Every loss taught me more about myself, my emotional triggers, and where my defenses were down. I learned to embrace the losses, seek God, fight on, and win.*

---

* Fred's book *Tactics: Securing the Victory in Every Young Man's Battle* (Colorado Springs, CO: WaterBrook, 2006) will help you deal with the emotional roots of masturbation. While part of a purity trilogy geared toward youth, *Tactics* can help any man of any age dump the masturbation.

10

Your Battle Plan 2: Accountability and a Band of Brothers

N ow that you have the outline of your battle plan, and before we focus in part 4 on the first of our three defense perimeters, let's take a brief look at a couple of special issues.

The first issue is accountability. For many men who are willing to fight for sexual purity, an important step is finding accountability support in a men's Bible-study group, in a smaller group of one or two other men serving as accountability partners, or by going to counseling.

For an accountability partner, enlist a male friend, perhaps someone older and well respected in the church, to encourage you in the heat of battle. The men's ministry at your church can also help you find someone who can pray for you and ask you the tough questions.

From Fred: Telling a Friend

But, Fred, you never had an accountability partner! That's true. No books had been written on the topic, churches hadn't yet developed the concept, and I was pretty certain that I was the only man in the entire state of Iowa struggling with this mess. It never crossed my mind to enlist another solid Christian guy to fight at my side. It was just the Lord and me out there alone on the battlefield.

Against all odds, I won anyway—not because I'm special but because God is special. So if you absolutely can't find an accountability partner, be encouraged. You can still win the battle. But please know that fighting alone is not your best option.

Oh, sure, I understand your sentiment: *I got this. I'm a man. I don't need anyone else.* You want to amble slowly out to the center of a dusty street at high noon and menacingly stare down the Enemy with your six-shooter at your side. You want to take on the world like some terminating cyborg and change history, all by yourself: *I'll grab this thing by the throat and smash it on my own.*

Listen, I understand rugged individualism very well, and I've lived it out on many fronts through the years. Succeeding on my own is at the core of who I am because it's rooted in my American culture.

There's certainly room for some of that attitude here. For one thing, if you want to win this battle, you do have to really want it as an individual. It's also crucial to form your own strong, internal defenses that require no one else's presence, especially since our culture is so sexually sick. Lastly, rugged individualism has its place in this battle because, in the final analysis, everything will come down to whether or not you've made a genuine decision to triumph here. Accountability works only when coupled with a firm personal commitment to win.

But the truth still remains that two are better than one in battle, and this is one more case where you need to be your own *apostolos* and insist that the culture of the Lord's kingdom supersede your own preferences. Jesus always sent His warriors into spiritual battle two by two. That is the kingdom pattern, and it must be your pattern here whenever possible.

I've heard all the arguments: *I don't want anyone else to know about my sin. It's embarrassing, and besides, I don't need another set of eyes looking over my shoulder like my mother. I'm an adult.* On its face, accountability can sound offensive. But if it does, it's probably because you have a limited understanding of the added strength that accountability offers.

For one thing, it provides a second set of eyes, which eliminates the secrecy that grants sexual sin much of its power over your life. Those eyes are also the reason the Covenant Eyes defense software is so potent and effective on your computer. You'll think twice before going to a porn site if you know an incriminating email will be sent to your buddy the moment you do so.

That's definitely a good thing because your warped synaptic patterns work on a use-it-or-lose-it basis, right? Every time you open a crass website, the dopamine reward strengthens your brain against you, but every time you avoid opening such a website, you weaken those pathways. If a second set of eyes keeps you from going to a porn site, why not invite that person in?

But the primary strength of accountability comes from the friendship and intimacy of the relationship and the insights shared together. Let me show you what I mean.

When my son Michael was training for his high school football team, we lifted weights extensively. I chose a nearby health club based on its weight room setup. The weight machines, which women tend to like, were all upstairs in a nice, well-lit, well-appointed room, while the free weights, which football players need, were all housed in a dimly lit underground bunker with ratty carpeting and cold cement block walls. Women rarely ventured there. Perfect.

As we prepared for Michael's sophomore season, he and I were lifting with some of his football buddies one night when three curvy teenaged babes in too-tight tank tops bounced into the room, giggling up a storm. They had no idea what they were doing with free weights and were clearly out of their element, but they sure had the guys' eyes popping out, practically telescoping like some real-life cartoon.

Michael kept his eyes where they belonged, of course, and neither of us said a thing about it until we were shuffling slowly across the parking lot after one more brutal workout. He was a step and a half behind me when I heard him say, "Dad, I don't think girls should be allowed to lift weights."

I chuckled hard, and he must have thought I misunderstood his meaning because he rushed to add, "Well, it's not that they aren't athletes and don't need to lift like the rest of us, but . . ."

I turned around and smiled. "It's because of what they were wearing, right, son?"

He looked as if I'd just dropped a coconut on his head. After taking a moment to regain his senses, he sputtered, "Yes, that's it exactly. Dad, don't they understand what they do to us when they dress like that?"

We tossed our gear into the trunk, and I stepped back to look him in the eye. "Son, sometimes they do understand and sometimes they don't, but I've learned that it really doesn't matter either way. What matters is what we do in response."

He nodded for me to continue. "I've discovered that a man cannot lust when using his peripheral vision, so this is what we're going to do the next time. While you're lifting, I'll keep track of where the girls are in my peripheral vision and I'll keep my back turned to them, and then when I'm lifting, you can keep track of them in your peripheral vision and keep your back to them. That way we'll be fine, whatever they wear. Sound good?"

He nodded again pensively as we climbed into the car. Firing up the engine, I turned onto Merle Hay Road and headed home. We drove without saying a word for a few miles, and then Michael broke our silence. "Thanks, Dad, for telling me about our peripheral vision. I'd have never thought of that on my own."

That's the power of accountability. Jesus didn't send His guys out two by two only so they would each have an extra pair of eyes looking over their shoulders; He sent them out with a brother so that they could learn from each other as they talked through the experiences of their day, just like Michael and me. The kingdom advances two by two far more quickly than one by one, and Michael's success on the battlefield advanced far more quickly than mine ever did on my own.

Accountability's Highest Power

The power of friendship and intimacy extends even beyond the sharing of tips and insights, as awesome as that is. If you think you don't need connection because you're a real man, we suggest that it is precisely *because* you are a real man that you need connection. As a red-blooded male, you have a weak spot in your sexuality that will always be open to attack when you're disconnected from others, no matter how strong your internal defenses feel today.

You see, it's not just the natural accountability in these relationships that gives connection its strength; it's the intimacy itself. You may think you don't need the accountability of those eyes in order to stand, but we can assure you, you *do* need the intimacy. It only makes sense that intimacy itself has the power to free you when you remember that our native language of intimacy is sexual, that masturbation feels like intimacy to us, and that porn and masturbation are like easily obtained feel-good drugs. Since masturbation provides a false intimacy that soothes emotional pain, our wounds and isolation have always left us open to this trap. You need *genuine* intimacy in your life to shut that trap permanently.

So, if you believe you don't need to get connected in accountability because you don't think you need a big Christian brother to stand with you in this fight or another set of eyes watching over your shoulder, you're missing the most important point. The primary goal of connection is to put genuine intimacy into your life so that it can replace the false intimacy you've been seeking through porn and masturbation. After all, who needs false intimacy when you have plenty of genuine intimacy in your life?

Amazing as it may sound, genuine intimacy is so potent that it can sometimes break the power of the masturbation cycle on its own. Will, a friend of mine, told me that a simple decision to get out of the house and connect with people broke the masturbation cycle when he was single:

I was always kind of a loner and stuck to myself a lot. Every night after work, I'd go home to my apartment all alone, and I'd wind up buried in pornography and masturbation. The experience left me feeling lonelier and more isolated! When friends at the office invited me places after work, or my family called to do things on weekends, I found myself saying no to all of them.

One day, I'd just had it with myself. Putting my foot down, I committed to saying yes to every invitation for the next four weeks, just to see what would happen. That was really hard at first because I felt out of place, like a third wheel. It was as though I had forgotten how to be with people in a casual environment. After a few experiences, however, I started getting comfortable and even loosening up around my friends and family.

Believe it or not, midway through the fourth week, I realized I hadn't masturbated in over ten days. A habit that had been with me for years began to fall away naturally as I reached out to other people. I won this battle without doing anything else but reaching out and connecting with others.

Essentially, Will went straight to the root of the problem and delivered the ax there by forming genuine intimacy in his life. You need accountability's powerful intimacy with you in the battle. Rich also found this to be true in his life:

I was very insecure as a child. Dad was distant because he worked a lot, so I bonded closely with my domineering, legalistic mother. Consequently, I never really felt like one of the guys. At school, I wasn't much of an athlete, so I played in the band. On top of that, my classmates tormented me, so I sought out masturbation to cope with the pain.

My porn and masturbation were never really about sex. It was about medicating pain and seeking emotional intimacy. Sometimes I think women view porn habits the same way they view the guys whooping it up at the strip club. They think it is all about lust and nothing more.

But it never was that way for me, and I really don't think it's that way for most of us. Masturbation was just my medication of choice. I could have easily gone the route of drugs or alcohol because the wounds at the root of the problem would have been the same no matter what substance I used.

But you know what eventually seemed to help the most in breaking this porn cycle? It turned out to be my best friend who really turned the tide for me. He was the first guy who truly accepted me as a man and as a friend. He affirmed my masculinity through our hiking adventures and our talks. Sometimes I think that a strong, masculine friend was all I needed.

Men need to be accepted as men, and Rich found freedom through the heart of a friend. It's intimacy between friends that makes accountability so crucial in this battle. This true intimacy and acceptance actually heals the underlying wounds, so the false intimacy of porn and masturbation is no longer necessary as a pain-killing medication in your life.

This is why wise Christian men are teaming up as "bands of brothers" in this fight. It isn't because they are weaklings; it is because they are smart. Sure, they might have to humble themselves by opening up to each other, but there has never been a time when that has been easier to do than today. Men all around the country are talking about the most embarrassing things, including masturbation, and because they are talking about these subjects, they are finding victory in the battle.

From Fred: Telling Your Wife

The accountability topic brings up the issue of how much you should tell your wife about your battle and how soon. As your understanding of your brain and your sexual habits grows, victory will seem more possible. With hope rising, perhaps you'll want to tell your wife about your battle for purity so that she, your dear, gracious wife, may help you win. But don't be in a big hurry.

Remember, our habits are rooted in our maleness. Because of that, *we* understand them. Women don't. Wives who learn of their husbands' struggles with impurity will often see them as betrayal, and they may see their husbands as perverts.

Some say that "right now" is always the best time to tell her. Well, I don't think it's an open-and-shut case, and in my defense, let me present Exhibit A.

Brenda and I were once discussing the fall of a prominent TV preacher to adultery. "If he were my husband," she stated, "I could not stand to even be around him. He would make me sick!"

Whoa. Brenda doesn't mince words, does she? But the plot quickly turned the next day when she broached the topic again. She told me she was feeling sorry for the disgraced preacher because he'd been desperately struggling alone against a secret sin. Brenda felt that if only his wife had known, she could have helped him through prayer.

"Fred," she said, "if you had such a problem, wouldn't you come to me and tell me? I would want to be praying for you and helping you!"

I burst out laughing. "Are you kidding me?" I replied incredulously. "Just yesterday you said you were totally repulsed by the guy. You'd cast me into a leper colony if I admitted such a thing!"

We laughed together, but this interchange highlights my stance perfectly. Women often swing between judgment and mercy, sometimes by the day, sometimes by the hour. The emotions run high, and it plays with your head on the battlefield.

That's probably why Brenda says the best time to bring your struggle up to your wife is *after* you've won the battle, which is the only genuine can't-miss proposition in this discussion.

It's in Your Court

We know that some men will disagree with us on this point. If you believe you ought to tell her immediately, that's fine with us because you know your own wife better than we do. It can work very well that way. We've seen many awesome wives swing directly to mercy and step right up to help their husbands on the spot. Perhaps your wife is one of these. Some wives even serve as their husband's accountability partner, and somehow that has worked too.

We caution you, however, against enlisting your wife as your full-blown, full-time accountability partner. There's no way most guys will get real with their spouses with something as starkly personal as one's thought life and masturbation habits, and there are even fewer wives who can stand the drip-drip-drip of your torturous admissions of failure over time.

For the most part, you just need to know that many wives react to sin with shock and revulsion at first rather than with mercy and prayer. We're just urging you to analyze your own situation carefully, especially in light of the following scenario.

How would your wife respond to you if she knew you had quit the battle, as you'll be tempted to do, especially in the first weeks? Before telling her, you had better check your will to win during the heat of battle. If you aren't yet sure you want to win, you'd be better off waiting to tell her because she'll be watching.

Brenda recently told me (Fred) that even now, all these years later, she occasionally watches my eyes when we go past billboards, just to check up on me. With the good habits in place, I haven't once failed her, but who needs that pressure if you aren't ready for it?

However, there *is* one thing we *can* say unequivocally: once you're absolutely sure that you hate your sin and you've begun to see positive changes in your life since engaging the battle, definitely tell your wife. Nothing is a better predictor of victory than a wife who willingly steps up to her husband's side in mercy, determined for both to come out stronger on the other end—together.

Since no one knows her husband better—his wounds, his stressors, his quirks— she'll be a priceless scout on the battlefield as he stretches to understand his own triggers and traps.

From Steve: Carefully, Prayerfully Decide When to "Tell All"

Having said all this, I want to add one more thing before we move on. During New Life's Every Man's Battle weekend workshop, we instruct guys to make a full disclosure to their wives as soon as possible. We emphasize the word *full* because you must get *all* the painful truth about your sin out on the table immediately. You may not feel ready to share all the details, but that's irrelevant. There must not be a dribble of new and painful information released over time because that's brutally selfish and self-defeating. It also inflicts a cruel, cyclical torture upon your wife.

Think about it. Every time she thinks she knows everything and begins to feel that she may be able to deal with it all, you dump another bucket of manure on her head. Bingo, she's right back in the painful sewer again. You may feel it's easier to get it out there little by little because of your embarrassment and shame, but you've been hiding and protecting yourself long enough. It's time to deal with this like a man. Protect *her* for a change. You made the mess, so *you* get it *all* out in the open and get the cleanup started.

It's also essential to consider the time and place that you make your full disclosure since there is a good chance that what you say will rip her heart out. Regardless of the condition of your relationship, it's not going to be easy for her to hear about your behavior. The pain will likely be unbearable early on.

Choosing to make a full disclosure on your own, therefore, can be a huge mistake. Even if you just want to get it all off your chest as soon as possible, I would strongly encourage you to consider telling her with a counselor or pastor in the room. This third party can help ensure that your wife hears exactly what you are saying and will be there to help her process and work through her initial shock from your revelation.

From Fred: Your Goal from Here

Now that you've made your decision for sexual purity, this is no time to retreat or second-guess yourself! You can see more than ever why failing to eliminate every hint of sexual immorality from your life is dangerous. The visual sensuality of immodest dress, movies, commercials, and all the rest will feed your eyes and ignite you sexually, and it will eventually misdirect your sexual neural pathways. The addictive nature of the chemical responses in your brain's pleasure centers spin tight cords of bondage.

To break those cords, you must cut off the sensual images through your eyes and mind. That's your goal, and the rest of the book is dedicated to showing you how to do it.

Level your sights on the Enemy, brother. It's time.

Part IV

Victory with Your Eyes

11

Bouncing Your Eyes

To set up your first defense perimeter around your eyes, you'll want to employ the strategies of bouncing your eyes and starving your eyes while using God's Word to take up a sword and a shield. We'll discuss each of these tactics in order over the next three chapters.

Let's first consider what we mean by bouncing your eyes. You can win this battle by training your eyes to bounce away from sensual sights in the women and images around you. If you bounce your eyes with consistency and determination for six weeks, you will develop a great habit that's critical in winning this war.

The problem is that your eyes have always bounced *toward* the sensual things in your environment and you've made no attempt to end this habit. It seemed natural because of the way your eyes are made, and since scoping out the female form is common among guys, it seemed harmless enough and just part of being a man.

But it isn't harmless, and this habit soon grows synaptic pathways that quickly transport these looks into pleasure highs. Because our culture is very sensual and our women often dress in tight and skimpy fashions, the highs hit often, the dopamine rewards hit hard, and before long, women become more of an interesting collection of body parts than daughters of the Most High God and our fellow heirs to the kingdom of grace.

In short, we end up objectifying women and see them as sex objects or potential sex partners, if not in real life, then at least in our minds and our fantasies.

To combat this effect and this habit, you need to build a reflex action by training your eyes to immediately bounce away from the sensual, like the jerk of your hand away from a hot stove.

Let's repeat that for emphasis: when your eyes become aware of a woman, you must train them to bounce away immediately. (Later, we'll explain how to handle bouncing your eyes with women you know.) Why must the bounce be immediate? After all, a glance isn't the same as lusting, right? If we define lusting as staring open-mouthed until drool pools at our feet, then a glance isn't the same as lusting. But if we define lusting as any look that creates that little chemical high, that little pop, then we have something a bit more difficult to measure.

Look, we know you can tell us whether or not you're drooling in lust. In fact, we can likely see it in your face or your eyes ourselves. But can you tell us exactly *when* that first look sends the impulse through your synaptic pathways and into the pleasure centers of the brain? That's a little more difficult to measure. This chemical high likely happens earlier in the process and much more quickly than you realize.

That's why, in our experience, drawing the line at "immediate" is clean and easy for the mind and eyes to understand. This line in the sand seems to work effectively.

So how do you train this new bouncing reflex until it becomes part of your daily experience?

For openers, the current habit of your eyes—focusing toward sensual things around you—is no different from any other habit. Since experts say that any action done consistently for twenty-one days becomes a new habit, our job is to give you a plan to consistently bounce your eyes *away* from the sensual over time, day by day, hour by hour.

From Fred: Your Tactics

When you begin bouncing your eyes, you can expect your body to fight against you in peculiar, unexpected ways, and you'll have to respond creatively. This is because sexual sin has an addictive nature, and your body will not want to give up on its pleasures.

Also, because your personal habits of sexual sin have their own unique flavor, your visual defense perimeter will have to be customized to your primary weaknesses to some extent. You'll customize your plan through these two logical steps:

1. *Study yourself.* How and where are you triggered visually the most? When it comes to your eyes, what are your biggest stumbling blocks out there?

2. *Define your defense.* You'll want to do this for each of the stumbling blocks you've identified.

Let's start out with that first step. Make a list of the most obvious and prolific sources of sensual images apart from your wife. Where do you look and lust most often? Where are you weakest?

To help you understand the process a little better, let me show how I originally customized my own battle plan. I had no problem coming up with a list of my six greatest areas of weakness. Keep in mind that my list predates the internet and smartphones:

1. Lingerie advertisements and magazine photo spreads
2. Female joggers in tight nylon shorts
3. Billboards showing scantily clad women
4. Beer-and-bikini commercials
5. Movies rated PG-13 or higher
6. Receptionists with low-cut or tight blouses

What are your main areas of weakness? In choosing them, remember that these must be areas from which you draw sexual satisfaction *visually.* Some guys aren't clear on this and make the mistake of choosing nonvisual weak spots for this list. For instance, Justin initially included the following three on his list:

1. Showers
2. Being home alone
3. Working late

We can all understand why these are troublesome. In the shower, you're nude with warm water cascading down your body. When you're home alone, no one is around to discover you. When you're working late, you feel sorry for yourself and need "comfort."

But remember, you're building a perimeter of the *eyes* here, so you have to be looking for the places where you take in *visual* sexual gratification from your environment so that you can train your eyes to bounce from and cut away this sexual pleasure at the source. This perimeter takes advantage of the use-it-or-lose-it life cycle of your synaptic pathways. If you cut the use of those pathways that you've developed over the years to handle your heavy visual sexual gratification, your mental train tracks will become less efficient in their processing. Eventually, the tracks will be torn up entirely.

Just so you understand, you don't have to directly attack these *nonvisual* weak spots like showers and working late. If you train your eyes to bounce and eliminate the visual stimuli, there'll be no food for the mental fantasies and sexual fever that draw your mind to sin in those situations. They are mere symptoms, not roots, and will lose their power over you naturally as you get your eyes under control.

Defining Your Defenses

Once you specify your greatest stumbling blocks, you'll need to define your defenses for each of them. While I can't determine the best defense for *your* weaknesses (since I don't know what they are), let me share how I defended my own so you'll get a feel for the process.

Catalogs and Magazines

Lingerie advertisements were my worst enemy and remained so for quite some time. I began successfully bouncing my eyes in the other five areas long before I had total victory here.

Why? Those ad inserts were the most sexually satisfying images of all for me, especially after I dropped the pornography from my life. From time to time, I'd hit the mother lode: a swimsuit feature or an exercise pictorial that was illustrated with bun-fitting spandex all around. I looked forward to my sessions with the Sunday morning newspaper like you might look forward to sessions of cyberporn.

Not only did I train my eyes to bounce away from such print ads, but I also trained myself not to pick them up in the first place. My defense was to establish a number of rules to keep these images out of my hands before my eyes had a chance to see them.

Rule 1: When my hand reached for a magazine or insert and I sensed in even the slightest way that my underlying motive was to see something sensual (rather than looking for a sale on tires or landscape timbers, for instance), I forfeited my right to pick up and peruse that week's ad insert, no matter what savings I might have discovered for our household budget.

To be honest, my new rule didn't work well at first: even though sensing my motives was easy, forfeiting my right to pick the ad up was not. My flesh simply ignored my spirit, shouting, *Shut up! I want this, and I will have it!* Sometimes I would win that argument and actually stand up and throw the ad inserts into the trash, but my brain would keep screaming for its high so loudly that I would return to the wastebasket ten minutes later, pull out the ads, take some satisfying looks, and masturbate. Finally, I started tossing cooked oatmeal remains or milk from my cereal bowl onto the insert after dumping it into the trash. That way it was nearly impossible for me to pull that insert back out to look at again.

As I began to succeed against those lingerie ad inserts, as well as in the other five areas, my hatred for the sin grew, and as it grew, my will and discipline grew stronger.

Rule 2: If a magazine had an overtly sensual female on the cover, I tore off the cover and threw it away.

Mail-order clothing catalogs and swimsuit magazines with sensual cover pictures can sit on your coffee table and draw your eyes all month long. Now, I ask you this: What if a full-breasted woman in a teensy-weensy bikini came to your home and sat down on your coffee table and said, "I'll just rest here for a couple of weeks, but I promise to leave by the end of the month"? Would you let her stay there to catch your eye every time you walked in the room for weeks on end? I don't think so. So why would you leave her there in picture form on the front of a magazine?

There were funny moments along the way. I remember a perplexed Brenda asking me one time, "What's been happening to all our magazine covers?" But that's how I handled the problem, and once I explained things to her, she happily granted me full censorship rights!

Rule 3: If I was genuinely looking for sale prices on camping equipment or tools in those department store inserts, I would allow myself to pick up the insert, but I forced myself to open it from the back.

Don't ask me how I knew, but the lingerie ads were usually found on pages 2 and 3 in these inserts. The camping, automotive, and tool ads were on the last pages. By opening the insert from the rear, I could search for sales while avoiding the hot young models up front.

When a sensual image snuck up on me even though my motives for leafing through a magazine or insert were proper, I kept the normal covenant to bounce my eyes immediately, and I would either tear out the offending page (so I wouldn't run across it again next time I picked up the magazine) or throw the magazine away.

Female Joggers

Whenever I approached a roadside jogger while driving my car and my eyes fixed on her, I'd soak up her beauty just as Steve did with the Malibu jogger he told of in chapter 1. But trying to look away from a jogger created a problem: I'd have to look completely away from the road not to see her. That was driving dangerously, even in Iowa!

Studying the situation, I found a solution. Rather than look completely away, I could simply look to the opposite side of the road. You see, as I creatively sought a solution, I discovered that it was impossible to lust with only my peripheral vision. Obviously, I immediately used that to my advantage with joggers, just as I taught Michael to do years later in the weight room.

But that didn't end my issues with joggers because my body began to fight back in interesting ways. First, my brain argued fiercely with me, saying, *If you keep this up, you'll cause a wreck. You'll certainly deserve prison when that happens!*

I considered this argument, but since my peripheral vision was now working in my favor, I sneered back, *You and I both know that's highly unlikely. You're just an addict squirming for your little high!*

It's important that you call things as they actually are in this battle to keep yourself from falling to deceit.

My body's second attempt to stop me was even more peculiar. Whenever I saw a jogger and reflexively looked away, my mind would trick me into believing I recognized the individual, prompting a second look. My mind was so good at this that before long, nearly every female jogger I saw reminded me of someone I knew.

Isn't that weird? It was as if every woman I knew had started jogging. You talk about irritating! It took a while for me to stop falling for that deception. My mind would snort, *Don't be so rude! When you know someone, you need to wave. You're a Christian, for heaven's sake!* I had to decide, for God's purposes, that it was more important for me to be rude and *not* wave at someone—whom I probably didn't know anyway—than it was to look more closely at her body to see if I recognized her.

My brain tried another trick. As I passed a jogger without a direct look, I would momentarily relax. I'd gloat, thinking, *Aha! I beat you that time!* But in that very same moment, my brain took advantage of my lowered guard and turned my eyes to glance into the rearview mirror for a more direct look. That really burned me up! I had to learn not to drop my guard after passing a woman successfully, and in time that trick faded away as well.

Whenever another brain trick worked, I'd bark to myself in sharp rebuke, *You've made a covenant with your eyes! You have no right to do that anymore.* In the first two weeks, I must have snarled that at myself hundreds of times, but the repeated confession of truth eventually worked to transform my mind.

Billboards

Billboards are notorious for featuring a long, tall, slinky, sexy woman who seems to whisper, "C'mon, big boy, buy this stuff and you'll get me too!" One rock radio station promoted their morning drive-time duo with a giant billboard that sported an enticing close-up of bikini-clad breasts with this tagline: "What a pair!"

My defense mechanism for billboards began with bouncing my eyes, of course, but I took it a step further by memorizing where the sensual billboards had been placed along my commute. That way I could look away earlier and ensure myself that I wouldn't drive up to them each day and get tomahawked.

When designing my billboard defenses, I thought of my experience in high school driving a hotel van. We had a contract with the airlines to drive pilots and flight attendants from the airport to the hotel. The contract required that we complete the trip within ten minutes. Only one route from the airport was short enough to make the time limit: an unpaved road with a billion potholes. I painfully learned of the direct correlation between the number of potholes I hit and the size of my tip. So I methodically memorized every pothole on that road and the driving angles necessary to miss most of them. Eventually, I could practically drive that road blindfolded and hit very few potholes.

With the billboards, it's always easier for me to memorize their locations and avoid visual contact entirely rather than to look at them first and then bounce my eyes.

Commercials

A red-blooded American male can't watch a major sporting event without being assaulted by commercials showing a bunch of half-naked women cavorting on a beach with some beer-soaked yahoos. What's a man to do?

The answer is to maintain control of the remote and use it as if it were a phaser or blaster to zap those commercials. The defense is simple: all sexy women get zapped by the clicker. *Phasers set to kill, Spock.* This is the best way. You can hit another station and come back in sixty seconds, or you can DVR your favorite sporting events and zip through the commercials—and those bikini-and-beach ads—and get right back to the game.

As your children watch you click away from or zip through the sensual ads, you serve as a living example of godliness in your home, and that will speak volumes to them. For instance, I'll never forget watching a Super Bowl one year with my boys when, during a commercial break, a full-screen close-up of a babe's bikini bottom splashed across the screen without warning. Michael instantly turned away and groaned heavily, but note this: he was only five years old at the time, and I'd never once talked to him about sensuality or bouncing his eyes.

How did he learn to turn from the screen with a groan? The answer: like any boy, he looked up to his dad and his thirteen-year-old brother, Jasen, and he wanted to be like us. We were a living example of godliness in his life, and he picked up on that naturally.

Movies

We had two very good media rules around the house when the kids were still living with us. First, if any video was unsuitable for children, it was probably unsuitable for adults. Second, if it polluted the landscape sexually, it didn't play. With these rules in place, sensual movies were never a problem in our home, and our boys never got carried away by sexual visuals that could have awakened their sexuality early and led them to porn and masturbation.

Not watching randy movies or roaming the internet is more difficult when you're on the road and in a hotel room all by yourself. Still, you want to be a real man who acts exactly the same when you're by yourself as when you're out in public, as well as a Christian who lives like a Christian when no one else is around.

Do you remember the transport device in *Star Trek* that made the phrase "Beam me up, Scotty!" part of the cultural lexicon? Your goal on any business trip is to live so honestly that your wife could "beam into" your hotel room at any moment and never find you watching or doing something improper.

With that standard in place, I would have been busted repeatedly earlier in my work life. Once five o'clock came around and the business day was over, I had hours ahead of me with nothing to do. This left me very vulnerable to watching cable movies, and I fell for them again and again.

So, to build out my defenses here, I set some ground rules. Whenever I reached for the remote, I would check my motives, just as I did with the ad inserts and magazines. If my motives were clean, I would allow myself to turn on the TV, usually sticking with cable news, ESPN's *SportsCenter,* or a football game. Trouble was, I would sometimes get bored and, without thinking, start channel surfing.

The "motive rule" worked better with magazines because once I forfeited the right to look at them, I could get up and go elsewhere and forget about them. Not so with the hotel room TV; I still had hours alone in the room with the blank screen staring back at me, tempting me.

So here's what I did: I simply grounded myself from hotel TV entirely. I decided that because of my bad behavior in the past, I'd lost my privileges and wasn't allowed to turn the TV on in any hotel room until I had broken all my bad habits.

Sound drastic? Not really. I've had some men tell me that they put blankets over their hotel TVs to keep them out of sight. I've had others say that they would regularly call ahead to the front desk and ask them to block the pay-per-view soft-core movies, while some even asked management to remove the television sets from their rooms before they arrived. Whatever you have to do, do it.

As for me, I began hauling along a truckload of extra office work and a couple of books to read at night, which kept my focus entirely off the TV and eventually allowed the offending synaptic pathways, which were built up over years of masturbation in hotel rooms, to wither and die. When the pathways were gone, my brain no longer tugged me in that direction. It has been decades since a television has tempted me in a hotel room.

Receptionists

Sometimes when I entered office buildings on sales calls, the receptionist would happen to be standing. After I told her my name, she would bend over to dial up my client to announce my arrival. Often her loose-fitting, silky blouse would fall open to reveal everything. In the past, it had never occurred to me to turn away; I simply figured it was my lucky day.

But once I began building a covenant with my eyes, this had to stop. The defense was simple. Whenever the receptionist was standing and she started to bend over to make that phone call, I'd avert my eyes toward the waiting area at my side, even before she bent over. Or if I saw her walking toward a file cabinet, I'd avert my eyes before she bent over for a file and left me a nice view of her rear end. Of all my visual stumbling blocks, this one was the easiest to overcome. I now habitually turn away without thinking about it at all.

The Internet

The internet wasn't in widespread use during my battle for purity, but if it had been, I'm absolutely sure it would have landed in my top trouble spots, just as I'm sure that accessing the World Wide Web will be in yours as you develop your own defenses. So let's talk about a defense strategy for the internet.

Obviously, software nannies are available to sift out the porn sites, and I recommend them as part of your overall strategy. But web pages—especially those that are the product of a search engine like Google—are loaded with all kinds of sensual thumbnail images to entice you to click on them. As you undoubtedly know, there is an endless display of racy photos, ads of busty women, and suggestive taglines to capture your eyes 24/7.

What do you do? Simply apply the same kinds of rules to your internet use that I applied in my battles, as I've explained above.

But, Fred, things are so much tougher out there today! You can't escape this stuff. It's everywhere!

One of the greatest lies you'll hear is that the broad impact of today's technology has turned today's battlefield into a muddy quagmire that you'll never escape. I understand the sentiment, but frankly, that's absurd.

Sure, it's true that your slippery slope is much steeper now because sexual content can be accessed on a broad range of platforms. It's also true that smartphones have placed pornography at your fingertips twenty-four hours a day and that today's streaming porn is far more violent and misogynistic than yesterday's static photo spreads seen in soft-core porn magazines at the local convenience store. I also understand that your sons and daughters, if they've hit the teen years or beyond, are viewing heavier sexual content on TV shows and films and on their iPads at earlier ages than mine did. Things *have* changed in access and content.

But things *haven't* changed when it comes to the hand-to-hand combat and self-defense necessary to win this battle. For instance, nothing has changed with your male eyes. Your eyes work exactly the same way as mine did years ago, and if you bounce them and starve them, you will cut off the outside sexual gratification that overhypes your sex drive and keeps you trapped in sin.

Nothing has changed with your brain and its chemistry either. Your addictions have grown by overstimulating and rewarding the neural pathways running to your pleasure centers, just as mine grew years ago. But they'll be eliminated when you go cold turkey on the dopamine and degrade the cords of synaptic connections through the same use-it-or-lose-it principle that has always governed neural real estate.

In short, your victory will still come through knowledge and discipline, regardless of the shifting tides or contours of the battlefield. Let me show you what I mean.

When it comes to the internet, for instance, you can start with my motive rule. When you power up the screen and your hand reaches for the mouse—and you sense in even the slightest way that your underlying motive is to see something sensual—shut down your computer or tablet instantly and walk away. Give yourself a break until you realign your mind with God's ways. It might be five minutes or it might be fifty minutes before you feel like you can hit the power button again, but that's okay.

The same sort of mind-set works for smartphones. If you look at your apps and decide to press on Google, Firefox, or "news" apps that are known for their tabloid fare and pictures of scantily clad women with the hope or expectation that you'll see something racy, turn off your smartphone for the same five minutes or until your mind is in the right place to turn your phone back on.

This new rule might not work well initially, even though sensing your motives is pretty easy. Forfeiting your right to keep the power on is *not* easy at first and, in fact, is rather challenging. Your flesh may try to ignore your spirit, shouting, *Shut up! I want this, and I will have it!* Or you may feel like you need to keep your smartphone on because someone could call you or send a text.

Sometimes you'll win that argument and actually stand up and walk away, but sometimes your brain will keep screaming so loudly for its high that you'll come right back to the computer or smartphone and fail miserably. That's okay. Get up and fight again, and remember that every time you *do* say no and power down, you'll weaken your warped synaptic pathways a little more and make the next "fistfight" easier.

You might install the two media rules that we Stoekers used around our house. If you see any sensual thumbnails or clickbait that looks too sensual for your kids, it is likely unsuitable for you. Don't click on it. Second, if that YouTube video looks like it might pollute the landscape sensually, don't hit Play. With rules like these in place, thumbnails and streaming videos lose their power over time. Remember, your goal is to live so honestly that your wife could "beam into" your smartphone, computer, or office at any moment and never find you watching anything improper.

Finally, I find my peripheral-vision principle to be quite helpful in my internet defenses. Sometimes I'll be scrolling down the screen on my computer and a thumbnail photo of a half-naked woman pops into view, but I've found a solution. Rather than look completely away from my screen, which can make it difficult to scroll away from the offending photo, I'll simply look to the opposite edge of my screen—away from the thumbnail.

Knowing that it's impossible to lust with my peripheral vision, I can immediately bounce my eyes away from the thumbnail and keep the image in my peripheral vision until I can scroll back up and away from the thumbnail. This happens dozens of times a day, and my little trick has become such a good, dependable habit that I don't even think about it anymore. The defense simply takes over automatically, just like a software nanny does with porn sites.

Remember, nothing has really changed at the core of this battle. Whether you're still going to the convenience store to pick up your porn or viewing it on your phone on the subway ride home, the battle's still the same. You must find ways to degrade the choking cords of your synaptic pathways by cutting away the sensuality that's flowing constantly into your eyes and brain. Go cold turkey on all of it, whatever it takes.

Some of this turnaround happens easily, like when you purchase good defense software. Some of this will be much more difficult, like when your pleasure centers are screaming for dopamine and you're screaming back in return, *No possible way! You can't have it!*

But that's what you have to do.

Every. Single. Time.

Moving On

So that's how you go about building defenses for the biggest visual stumbling blocks in your life. But it doesn't stop there. As you're dealing with those, you'll continue building out your visual defense perimeter by embracing a concept we'll explore in the next chapter: starving your eyes.

12

Starving Your Eyes

A s you continue laying a defense perimeter into place around your eyes, a further strategic approach is to think in terms of starving your eyes. Remember again our definition for sexual purity: you are sexually pure when you're getting no sexual gratification from anyone or anything but your wife. Victory requires starving out all sexual gratification delivered through the eyes except that which involves your wife.

Here's another way to picture that gratification. As a man, you're used to consuming a certain amount of food and water each day. The amounts differ for each of us and are based upon our habits, genetics, metabolism, and activity. It's possible to suspend these needs for a while, as when you're fasting or limiting your food intake to lose weight. With some will and effort, you can get used to consuming fewer calories permanently by consistently cutting the amount you take in each day.

Similarly, you have been used to getting a certain amount of sexual gratification each day, some from your wife and some through your eyes. You can adjust your intake and get used to a lower daily volume of sexual gratification. With some will and effort, you can starve out the sexual images entering through your eyes and your mind's eye, and your body will become used to living on less.

Bowls of Gratification

Unfortunately, there's no unit of measure, like liters or inches, for sexual gratification. But we're going to make one up, and we'll call them bowls. Imagine that your current level of sexual hunger takes in about ten bowls of sexual gratification per week. These bowls of pleasure should be filled from your single legitimate vessel of sexual fulfillment, the wife God provided for you. But because we can soak up sexual gratification through our eyes, we can effortlessly fill our bowls from other sources.

Our sensualized culture pours out sexual imagery freely with the potential to fill our bowls continually and forever. Our eyes can feast away! If your current sexual hunger is at ten bowls a week and your wife is serving up only five, you can easily draw five bowls from the culture around you. (That's not the same as having intercourse with our wives five times a week because we can draw sexual gratification from our wives in many ways.)

While this bowl imagery oversimplifies the details, it clarifies the process involved in satiating our sexual hunger.

From Fred: Starving Your Eyes

To attain sexual purity as we defined it, you must starve your eyes and phase out the bowls of sexual gratification coming from outside your marriage. When you starve your eyes and eliminate "junk sex" from your life, you'll deeply crave "real food": your wife. And no wonder. She's the only thing in the kitchen cabinet, and you're hungry!

After slamming my fists into the steering wheel on Merle Hay Road and engaging the battle to build a covenant with my eyes, I began starving my eyes in earnest. If you remember my story, what I wanted most was the ability to look God in the eye again in prayer, with the added hope that I might finally be able to connect intimately with Him in worship as well. I did not think that starving my eyes would have even the slightest direct impact upon my deep connection with Brenda or my sexual relationship with her. I already had a very satisfactory sexual relationship with her, and I didn't figure our connection could be much better either. Boy, was I mistaken.

I began starving my eyes with a vengeance, and not just in the weakest arenas that I listed in the previous chapter. Visually, I slashed every sensual thing out of my life. I stopped watching women's ice skating and women's beach volleyball competitions. I stopped watching the early morning exercise shows on television. I even stopped daydreaming of busty women I saw at work or thinking about old girlfriends in sensual ways in my mind's eye. I dumped every last little thing that might rush some sexual gratification into the pleasure centers of my brain via the synaptic tracks.

I was stunned at what happened about two weeks into it. I remember vividly how Brenda began looking like a supermodel to me. Even my wife noticed the geometric rise in my desire for her. I was constantly telling her how beautiful she looked, and I was all over her, patting her, hugging her, touching her. I also was desiring intercourse far more often.

Sure, I'd always found her attractive, but whoa—now I couldn't keep my eyes off her. I began saying things to her that I hadn't uttered for years, quick asides like, "Man, you are *so* hot," or "I can't wait for tonight, baby." All my imaginative creativity was now blossoming upon our marriage bed, not in some fantasy world. I was fully enamored with her!

I didn't quite know what was happening, and at first I didn't connect the dots between starving my eyes and this new view of Brenda. She didn't know what was happening either, but I can assure you of one thing: she was not amused.

Let's face it: anyone who's been married for a while knows that couples eventually find an equilibrium when it comes to sex. In other words, on Sunday night you pretty much know how many times you'll have sex by the following Saturday. There's a pattern and you both know the drill.

But by starving my eyes, I'd upset the equilibrium. Until then, I'd been getting perhaps five bowls of gratification from Brenda each week, primarily through physical foreplay and sexual intercourse. I'd also been getting five bowls from outside my marriage, through foreplay of my eyes and masturbation.

Things had been at equilibrium for both of us, but Brenda had been accustomed to providing me only five bowls a week. The trouble was, I was still hungering for ten, and so now I was suddenly soliciting the extra five bowls from *her* that I used to get *outside*.

She didn't know I was starving my eyes. All she knew was that I was now calling for intercourse twice as often, for absolutely no apparent reason to her. This new-found hunger shocked her.

Oh, sure, she knew that men always want more sex than they're getting. But to her, there seemed to be more to this. And there was! Since my visual gratification now poured only from her, she was looking very good to me. I hadn't looked at her quite like that since we were newlyweds. While that sensation was vaguely pleasant to her, it was also jarring.

She later told me that many questions ran through her mind during those days. *Has he found an aphrodisiac?* she wondered. She didn't quite know what to do about that if I had, except to send me outside to play with the kids whenever she was showering and getting ready for the day or changing clothes in the master bathroom.

She also wondered if I'd been having an affair. *He's been telling me how hot I am and patting me all the time. Is he having an affair and covering his tracks with all this extra affection? What's going on here?*

She figured the most likely cause was something like the food jags she had during pregnancy, when she couldn't eat enough Hostess Ding Dongs. *Perhaps Fred's itch for me is like that jag and it will be over soon. I certainly hope so!*

Putting Up with Me

After a couple more weeks of starving my eyes, nothing had changed, and as the new higher pace of my hunger showed no sign of abating, it dawned on Brenda that this might not be just some simple jag or a phase. It might be permanent!

She began to panic, and the next time I wandered into the kitchen and ogled her body with a low whistle, she whipped around and leveled a finger at me, blurting, "Tell me what I am doing to be so attractive so I can stop it!"

That moment—and the fierce glare on her face—was hilarious. But also in that moment, everything came together and connected the dots in my mind. I told her what was going on and how I was starving my eyes and that I couldn't help my heightened desire for her at that moment.

"All my desires are coming straight at you, and I don't quite know what to do about it yet," I said. "I promise I'll work hard to get back to an equilibrium that we both can live with."

Brenda didn't know whether to be relieved or shocked, but when I explained that I was doing all this for the sake of our family and to crush the generational sin in my line, she was all in. She expressed a willingness to allow me time to find that equilibrium and to put up with me until then.

Those days revealed to me just how much I'd been stealing from Brenda by watching sensuous R-rated movies, inspecting the lingerie catalogs, and gawking at joggers in sports bras. Those things provide far more sexual gratification than you might expect, although Satan would have you think otherwise.

When a fellow named Tom heard me speak about removing every hint of sexual sin from our lives, he said, "I think you're defining sexual sin much too broadly when you include movies, ad inserts, joggers, and the rest. Those are little things. They're nothing!"

I disagreed, and why not? I was evidently drawing so much sexual gratification from these "innocuous" sources that once they were removed and the whole sexual burden was placed upon Brenda, she felt it herself. These are hardly little things, especially if they can transform how you view your wife.

A Quick Word to Single Men

Before we move on, let's freeze-frame this moment and note that it's also important for single guys to understand just how much sexual gratification is gained from these "little things." If you want to get your sexual desires under control, you can't expect to consume this many bowls of gratification from the outside world without driving your sexual engines well past the redline and into masturbation.

But how am I ever going to find a marriage partner if I'm starving my eyes of women all the time?

Without a doubt, this is the most frustrating question we receive from unmarried readers because it reveals a misunderstanding of sexual purity. Starving your eyes doesn't mean you must walk across your school campus staring at the concrete and avoiding the eyes of every girl you meet. That would be ludicrous, and it would defeat the entire purpose of purity, which is to restore our interaction with women to a natural, healthy, and innocent state.

We're not saying that you can't have any female friends or have any close connection to women anymore. You absolutely should have tons of female friends, and you'll definitely relate closely to women in church and in business for the rest of your life. So, when we advise you to starve your eyes, we're not suggesting that you flee from women or be nervous around them. Quite the opposite.

One time during his college years, I asked my son Jasen how he kept his eyes and heart pure at Iowa State University when there were many attractive coeds in too-tight tank tops and shorts. "After all, you can't ignore them, right?" I queried.

"No, and I wouldn't want to," he replied. "I'm friends with a lot of girls, especially since I'm a campus ministry leader now. I've just decided to deal with girls from the neck up, Dad. That way, we can talk and joke and laugh and have a great time, but it still feels very natural. It works perfectly for my purity too, probably because when we're relating to each other from the neck up, their bodies are always down there, somewhere in the safety zone of my peripheral vision. If they aren't dressed as modestly as I would like, it still never becomes a problem for me."

Jasen got it, didn't he? Starving your eyes is meant to free you when you're around women, not chain you. It's meant to remove any low-grade sexual fevers you might feel around women because of the way you've objectified them in the past. Clearly, Jasen felt comfortable around girls, and they, in turn, felt safe and comfortable around him. Girls weren't just an interesting collection of body parts to him, and they knew it.

Let me assure you, in that kind of healthy environment, you'll have no problem finding a wonderful young woman for life, even while starving your eyes.

And now, let's get back to my story with Brenda.

Adjusting to Purity

Brenda and I did eventually find that new sexual equilibrium. My sex drive was retooled to live within God's boundaries, but it didn't happen until I went cold turkey and deprived myself of impure sexual images from outside my marriage.

Am I still getting the full ten bowls of sexual gratification every week? Nope, but I haven't dropped all the way to five either. Brenda still provides extra bowls through an increased frequency of sexual intercourse and other related fun, but there's also been a natural downward adjustment of my sexual hunger, maybe dropping from ten bowls to six or seven a week as I adjusted to my new sexual purity.

Wait a minute, Fred, you say. *Cutting down from ten bowls to six bowls seems unfair. If I follow your path, I'll be cheated sexually, all because I'm obeying God!*

I guarantee you won't feel cheated. First, without the constant hyperstimulation of your sex drive from visual binging, your sexual hunger will return to normal, original specs. Second, with your whole sexual being now focused on your wife, sex with her will be so transformed that your satisfaction will explode off any known scale, even while consuming fewer bowls. It's a personal guarantee, backed by the full faith, credit, and authority of the Word of God.

Still Beautiful

We think Liam's story can help deepen your understanding of this paradox. Speaking of his wife, Regina, he told us that things got to the point where she just didn't excite him anymore. He said, "What with the chaos of parenting and year after year of being responsible for the kids, Regina had become just a good, trusted friend. She always came through in the clutch, but like any good friend, I didn't find her particularly sexy.

"Then one day, I was making a delivery in a building downtown and, rounding a corner, I came face to face with a goddess. Young, with long, rich black hair. Long legs in heels and full breasts crowning a silky-thin, miniskirt sundress. I actually gasped out loud. It was totally embarrassing. My chest heaved, and my mouth instantly went bone dry. I may or may not have staggered—I don't know. But I felt as if I'd been knocked cold.

"From time to time over the next few days, I got to thinking about Regina as I drove around at work. My wife had never been jaw-dropping beautiful, even when younger. I remembered, though, that when I first laid eyes on her, she was very striking to me and blew all my whistles! I wondered, *Is she still beautiful to me?*

"One night, as I watched her prepare dinner for us, I noticed that she was still quite pretty. She was a bit heavier, and her rear end hung a little, as did the skin around her eyes and neck. But she was pretty to me. *Why don't I appreciate her beauty anymore?*

"Shortly after that, I heard Fred speak about starving your eyes. I'd never been in gross sexual sin, but I'd never really guarded my eyes either. I watched any movies I wanted, and I often looked a little too long at the younger girls at work, yet I really didn't think these things affected my life. But after Fred's talk, I began to wonder. I paid more attention to my eyes, and I found that they were collecting a lot more sexual gratification than I'd thought.

"Thinking maybe that was why I'd lost my appetite for Regina, I began starving my eyes. I couldn't believe what happened! Regina is no longer just a friend; she's become a goddess, at least to me. And it's funny—the more I draw from only her, the more my tastes change. Those little rolls of fat on her back and sides used to bother me. Now as I run my fingers over them, they actually turn me on. Isn't that crazy? And that little bit of rear end that hangs below her underwear? Before, it only emphasized to me how much weight she'd gained. Now that little piece just explodes my desire for her. Regina may not be a supermodel, yet to me she's like Miss America."

The Sexual Payoff

The magazines at the supermarket checkout might say, "Fantasize to a Better Sex Life." The talk shows may say, "Let variety improve your sex life—adultery can be good!" But in God's kingdom, obedience always ends in joy and peace—and, in this case, thrills.

You can count on a sexual payoff from obedience. Proverbs 5:18 says, "May your fountain be blessed, and may you rejoice in the wife of your youth." Whether your wife is wide or narrow or lumpy or smooth, when you focus your full attention on "your fountain," she'll become ever more beautiful to you. Her weak points will become sexy because her body is yours and yours alone. Her characteristics are what you have, so you can cherish them and let them fulfill you.

Maybe this shouldn't surprise us so much. After all, standards of beauty are not fixed. In centuries past, the great master painters depicted heavy, rounded women as the ultimate beauty. In the 1920s, thin, flat-chested women reigned. In the 1960s, the full-breasted, voluptuous girls were queen. In the 1980s and 1990s, muscled, glistening athletic women ignited us. Presently, women with humongous fake breasts and Botox have moved into favor. Men adapt to each time period, their tastes formed by what they view and by whom they have sex with.

If you limit your eyes to your wife only, your own tastes will adapt to what you're viewing. Your wife's strengths and weaknesses will become your tastes. Eventually, she'll be beyond comparison in your eyes.

13

Your Sword and Shield

These strategies for bouncing and starving your eyes may sound rather simple, maybe even easy to do, but they aren't.

Satan fights you with lies while your body fights you with the desires and strength of deeply entrenched bad habits and synaptic pathways. To win, you need a sword and a shield. Of all the parts of your battle plan, perhaps these are the most important.

Your Sword

You'll need a good Bible verse to use as a sword and rallying point.

Just one? It may be useful to memorize several verses of Scripture about purity, as they work to eventually transform and wash the mind. But in the cold-turkey, day-to-day fight against impurity, trying to use several memory verses at once might be as cumbersome as strapping on a hundred-pound backpack to engage in hand-to-hand combat. You aren't agile enough.

That's why we recommend a single attack verse, and it had better be quick. We suggest the opening line of Job 31:

I made a covenant with my eyes.

When you fail and look at a jogger, say sharply, *No, I've made a covenant with my eyes. I can't do that!* When you look at a busty billboard, say, *No, I've made a covenant with my eyes. I can't do that!* This action will be a quick dagger to the heart of the Enemy. It is Scripture, after all, and it is the new reality you are training into your brain.

Your Shield

Your shield—a protective verse that you can reflect on and draw strength from even when you aren't in the direct heat of battle—may be even more important than your sword because it helps eliminate temptation and moves it out of earshot. We suggest selecting these verses as your shield:

> Flee from sexual immorality. . . . You are not your own; you were bought at a price. Therefore honor God with your [body]. (1 Corinthians 6:18–20)

We've distilled this shield verse to its core kernel and repeated it in the face of many tempting situations when facing sensual images or thoughts: *You have no right to look at that or think about it. You haven't the authority.*

A shield such as this will help you think rightly about the real issues involved as you face temptation in your fight for purity. Satan's power of temptation lies in your *supposed* right to make decisions regarding your behavior. If you understand clearly that you no longer have the right to make these choices, the Enemy's tempting power can't touch you because he's never invited into the conversation. In this way, you neutralize the Deceiver's voice in your life.

From Fred: Looking at *Playboy*

Once on an overnight hotel stay, I walked down the hallway to the ice machine. On top of the machine was a *Playboy* magazine. Mistakenly believing that I had a right to choose my behavior, I asked myself this question: *Should I look at this* Playboy *or not?*

The moment I asked that question, I opened myself to outside counsel. Sure, I began talking the pros and cons to myself internally, just as my question would suggest. But without noticing it, that question *also* opened me up to Satan's counsel. He wanted to be heard on this issue.

He cajoled and lied, keeping my mind focused on the conversation so I didn't even notice my body slipping down the slope of lust. By the time he'd finished, the only answer I wanted to hear myself say was, *Yes, you can look at it.*

Therein lies the power of temptation. We may fear that temptation will be too strong for us in this battle, but temptation honestly has no power at all without our own arrogant questions and the supposed right to choose our behavior. Once we become Christians, we are no longer to have such choice.

Now put yourself in my situation that night. Away from home on a business trip, you're walking to fill your ice bucket and you spy the *Playboy* magazine. But your mind has been dwelling upon your shield verse, the words from 1 Corinthians 6:18–20.

What's your internal response now?

I have no right to even consider looking at it. I haven't the authority. Christ owns me now.

Once that conviction is set firmly in place, it leaves no room for pros and cons to drift deceitfully through your brain. You get your ice and leave the magazine with no further thought. And as for Satan, since you asked no questions, no conversation with him transpires—a conversation in which he would definitely try to get you to change your mind.

We call this better response living within your rights. If you live within your rights, God's laws of reaping and sowing will protect you. Once you step beyond your rights, the sowing and reaping laws will work against you because you're in mutiny, having stolen authority from your Captain. And you're back within earshot of Satan. Shield yourself from the power of temptation by submitting to God's truth regarding your rights.

From Fred: What to Expect in the Short Term

Okay, let's say you've made a covenant to starve your eyes and to train them to bounce. You've defined your weak areas, creating a custom defense for each one, and have picked up your sword and shield. What can you expect to happen over the next few weeks? Here's a bit of the time line that unfolded for me as my perimeters went up.

The first two weeks were largely failure after failure for me. My eyes simply would not fall in line and bounce away from the sensual, and my mind's synaptic pathways clutched and clawed for their drugs. My shields from Satan's lies were also weak and flimsy, but I kept plodding ahead in faith, knowing God was with me.

During the third and fourth weeks, hope dawned as I began to win about as often as I failed. I can't overemphasize how dramatic and surprising this change was for me. God's blessings and gifts truly go beyond what we can ask for or imagine because, when we sow righteousness, only the mind of God can conceive of the blessings we'll reap. Already I couldn't believe how much I now lived to please Brenda.

During the fifth and sixth weeks, my eyes found a consistency in bouncing away from the sensual. At the end of the sixth week, I had the intense dream I spoke of earlier that opened me up to a new world of worship and intimacy with Christ. The spiritual oppression lifted, and the veil of distance from God vanished. Though I was still not perfect, the rest of my battle would be like a downhill ride by comparison.

The point is, it doesn't matter how long you've been tormented by sexual sin. It needn't take long to raise the defense perimeter of your eyes. If you really desire victory, it will come quickly. More than once, men have said to me, "Fred, this is amazing, but it happened just like you said! Right about the sixth week, it all came together!" But six weeks is surely no hard-and-fast rule. It may take more time, depending upon your strongholds and your commitment level to the task at hand.

However long it takes for you, persistence will be your best friend because of the use-it-or-lose-it nature of your addictive synaptic pathways. You have to *stop using* them to *lose* them, and there's only one way to stop using them: by persistently and consistently starving and bouncing your eyes.

From Steve: Have Realistic Expectations

I want you to know that too often men engage in this battle and expect to see immediate, radical victory over sexual temptation. When all the urges don't instantly die, their sense of shame and inadequacy sets them up for a severe relapse.

Please be realistic as you engage this battle. Approach it as if you're at the controls of a massive powerboat tearing through the waves. You may kill the engines, but you'll never stop in place. All the forces within and without are still in motion.

Your lust works the same way. You can cut your sexual engines, but there will still be some drift after choosing integrity. Accepting this up front makes it much easier to stay the course when things don't go as planned.

What to Expect in the Long Term

As you continue to live purely, the hedge of protection from temptation grows thicker around you. If you're diligent, Satan has a much longer throw if he wants to lob temptation grenades into your living quarters. In time, the synaptic pathways break down and your temptations weaken further.

In the long term, then, do you still have to monitor your eyes? Yes, because the natural bent of your eyes is to sin, and you'll return to bad habits if you're careless. But with only the slightest effort, good habits are permanent.

On a practical note, if you live in a four-season region, late spring and early summer call for a fresh dose of diligence, as warmer temperatures allow women to wear less clothing. Plan to heighten your defenses at those times.

After a year or so—though it may take longer—nearly all major skirmishes will stop. Bouncing your eyes will become deeply entrenched. Your brain, now policing itself tightly, will rarely slip anymore, having given up long ago on its chances to return to the old days of pornographic pleasure highs.

How difficult does this remain over time? It's up to you. The best picture we can draw is that of the Israelites' move into their Promised Land. They were promised a land of milk and honey where they would be at rest from their enemies.

But just like it was for the Israelites, you won't possess that place of peace without a fight, and you won't take that Promised Land without doing exactly what God says about destroying every trace of your old habits, as well as every belief about your so-called rights and freedom to look. Whatever you leave alive and don't destroy becomes mixture in your life, and it then becomes a snare to you. So take responsibility for your purity. Stand up and fight the right way.

Slightly Crazy?

Looking back at the details of our plan for your eyes, even we will admit that it all sounds slightly crazy. Defenses, brain tricks, bouncing your eyes, forfeiting rights. Man! We wonder if even Job would be a bit startled.

On the other hand, maybe we should expect a sound plan to look this way. Consider all the men who are called to purity, yet so few seem to know how to make it happen.

What's the bottom line? It took all our resources and creativity to destroy the old habits and every inch of freedom in Christ to walk free from sin. We had been owned by these habits for years, taking whatever women we desired with our eyes.

Freedom from sin is worth dying for, according to Jesus. Take it from us—it's also worth living for!

From Fred: Finding Purity Requires Commitment

A few years ago, an Iowa State University student, a Christian guy, stopped my daughter Rebecca in her dorm hallway and said, "I've read your dad's book, but I don't believe that *all* men are capable of walking purely when it comes to sensual things. Only some are given the grace to do so."

Well, anyone can cop an opinion, and that's his belief. But it's not the truth. It isn't a lack of *grace* that dooms us (see 2 Peter 1:3–4); it is a lack of *commitment* from us to build our defense perimeters and to stand up and fight. As guys, we simply haven't chosen to learn to control our bodies in holy and honorable ways, even though it's clearly God's will for us to do so (see 1 Thessalonians 4:3–4).

Are you ready to keep learning? Let's move on to part 5 and study further how to control our bodies by layering in a second defense perimeter, this time around our minds.

Part V

Victory with Your Mind

14

Your Mustang Mind

A s you build your outer defense perimeters, you'll find that the perimeter of the eyes goes up much faster than the perimeter of the mind. Why is that?

First, the mind is far craftier than the eyes and more difficult to corral. Second, you really can't rein in the mind effectively until the defense perimeter of the eyes is in place. You have to stop the flow of visual gratification to get control of your thoughts. Knowing this, you shouldn't be discouraged if your mind responds more slowly than your eyes.

The great news is that the defense perimeter of the eyes works with you to build the perimeter of the mind. The mind needs an object for its lust, so when the eyes view sexual images, the mind has plenty to dance with. Without those images, the mind has an empty dance card. By starving your eyes, you starve your mind as well.

But this alone is not enough, as the mind can nimbly create its own lust objects using memories of movies or images you saw years ago or by generating fantasies about old girlfriends or the women you work with. However, at least with your eyes under control, you won't be overwhelmed by a continuing flood of fresh lust objects pouring in as you struggle to learn to control your thoughts.

Your Mind Coming Clean

Currently, your brain moves nimbly to lust and to the little pleasure high it brings. Lustful thinking is your brain's guiding worldview. Double entendres, daydreams, and other creative forms of sexual thinking are approved pathways of thought in most everyone around you, so your mind feels free to run on those pathways to pleasure.

But it doesn't have to be that way. Your cultural mind-set and your worldview color what comes through the filters in your mind, and you can change those. This is important to know because your mind is orderly. The mind will allow these impure thoughts only if they fit the way you look at the world. As you set up the perimeter of defense, your brain's worldview will be transformed by a new matrix of allowed thoughts, or what we call allowables.

Within the old matrix of your thinking, lust fit perfectly and in that sense was orderly. Your brain did nothing on its own to arrest it. But with a new, purer matrix firmly in place, lustful thoughts will bring disorder. Your brain, acting as a responsible police officer, will soon learn to nab these lustful thoughts even before they rise to consciousness. While that may seem impossible for you to imagine right now, it's true. In short, the brain will eventually begin cleaning itself on a subconscious level so that elusive enemies like double entendres and sensual daydreams, which are hard to control on the conscious level, simply vanish from your daily experience.

This transformation of the mind takes some time as you wait for the old sexual pollution to be washed away. It's much like living near a creek that becomes polluted when a sewer main breaks upstream. After repair crews replace the cracked sewage pipe, it still takes some time for the water downstream to clear.

Sure, you'll be taking an active, conscious role in capturing rogue thoughts as you build a perimeter around your mind, but in the long run, the mind will wash itself and begin to work naturally *for* you and your purity by capturing such thoughts *before* they even arise. That is what transformation means! With the eyes bouncing away from sexual images and the mind policing itself, your defenses will grow incredibly strong.

Lurking at the Door

With that confidence, you'll want to be doing all you can to push along your mental transformation. A helpful concept in this regard is the scriptural imagery of "lurking at the door." Job mentioned it just a few verses after he discussed the covenant he made with his eyes:

If my heart has been enticed by a woman,
   or if I have lurked at my neighbor's door,
then may my wife grind another man's grain,
   and may other men sleep with her.
For that would have been wicked,
   a sin to be judged. (Job 31:9–11)

Have you "lurked at your neighbor's door"? It could mean stopping by in the late afternoon and visiting your friend's wife for coffee. Perhaps you're enamored by her wisdom, care, and sensitivity. Or maybe you've felt sorry for her as you've commiserated together over her insensitive, brutish husband. You've held her as she cried. If so, you were lurking at your neighbor's door.

Consider Kevin, who is married with three kids. While working with the youth group at church, he met a beautiful fifteen-year-old girl.

"She's a knockout and looks more like twenty," he said. "Sometimes I'd ask her about boys she's known and dated, and we'd joke and laugh a lot, but sometimes I went too far. We'd get to talking a little trashy about what she liked when kissing, what I bet she wouldn't do with a guy—that sort of thing. I knew I shouldn't talk to her like that, but it was exciting.

"Last week, when my wife and kids were out of town, I gave this girl a ride home. We got to talking dirty again, and before I knew it, I bet her that she wouldn't pull her pants down for me. She did. I lost my senses, and I drove her to a park and we had sex. I'm in real trouble! She told her parents about it, and they may press rape charges!"

That's the trouble with lurking at a neighbor's door: it so easily leads us past the threshold and into situations and sin we would never have believed ourselves capable of. In this case, a vulnerable young woman was violated and, ultimately, multiple lives were shattered.*

---

* Kevin (not his real name) was reported to the authorities for his actions, and he was sent to prison.

Mental Lurking

Maybe you've never done what Kevin did but you've been lurking at your neighbor's door just the same. According to Jesus, doing it mentally is the same as doing it physically (see Matthew 5:28).

You know you've lurked. Your friend's wife seems more like your type than your own wife. *Why didn't I meet her sooner?* you wonder. *How different things would have been if I had!* You're lurking.

Maybe your old girlfriend is married now, yet you lurk at her door in your mind, wondering if she misses you, secretly hoping to run into her at the mall or the grocery store.

Or you've been lunching with a group at work, including that beautiful young sales associate, getting so attached that you're depressed whenever she calls in sick. The last time she was absent, you sent her a warm email saying, "I missed you today . . . hope you feel better soon."

Maybe you've connected with a woman online and you imagine what life with her would be like and how it would feel to hold her. You're lurking at your neighbor's door.

Wild Thinking

As we've seen when discussing the perimeter of the eyes, most of your outside sexual gratification is generated by women you don't even know. You view them in passing. Models, actresses, receptionists, and online images are everywhere. But they're strangers. You never talk to them and your orbits don't cross daily at work or in the neighborhood, so training your eyes to bounce away is enough to defend yourself.

But bouncing your eyes cannot screen out those live attractions arising from actual social interaction with women. These women aren't strangers. You live and work in close proximity with them, even worshiping with them on Sunday. Impure thoughts and attractions may arise, and since the defense perimeter of the eyes won't work in these situations, you need another method of defense.

"What am I supposed to do?" you ask. "Those thoughts come on their own. I can't help them." That certainly *seems* true since you've never tried to control your mind, and your thoughts seem to race in out of the blue. Even in church, a sensual daydream may suddenly transpire about some woman at work. Where do these thoughts come from? The mind is like a wild mustang, running free, one thought triggering another in no real order. Still, the Bible says we are responsible to control not just our eyes but our entire bodies as well:

> You are not your own; you were bought at a price. Therefore honor God with your [body]. (1 Corinthians 6:19–20)

That includes your mind. The Holy Spirit, through Paul, is clear on this:

> We demolish arguments and every pretension that sets itself up against the knowledge of God, and we take captive every thought to make it obedient to Christ. (2 Corinthians 10:5)

This is a jarring verse. *Take every thought captive? Is that really possible?*

Your Mental Customs Station

It *is* possible, and it isn't as complex as one might think. All impure thoughts are generated as we process both visual and live attractions through our senses. Viewing women on the beach. Flirting with the new woman at work. Remembering an old girlfriend. If we improperly process these, our minds can get carried away in impurity. However, by properly processing these attractions, we can capture or eliminate impure thoughts.

We've already discussed one form of proper processing called bouncing your eyes. When it's effectively established, your defense perimeter of the eyes has the nature of the old Berlin Wall. No visual entry visas are ever granted for any reason.

But the defense perimeter of the mind is less like a wall and more like a customs

area in an international airport. Customs departments are filters, preventing dangerous elements from entering a country. The defense perimeter of the mind works in
a similar way by properly processing attractive women into your "country" while
filtering out the alien seeds of attraction before the impure thoughts are even generated. This perimeter stops the lurking.

Consider the situations of two men we've talked about. Wally, the businessman
who dreaded being alone in hotel rooms, found out that even after turning off the
TV, his mind still raced with sexual images in circle after circle of lustful bombardment until he couldn't sleep at all. Had he not granted *visual* entry visas by watching
TV, no lustful thoughts would have been dropped on him. The situation is different
for live attractions. Kevin was a youth-group *leader*, and that fifteen-year-old girl
was a youth-group *member*. She had a valid entry visa into his life, and there was
no Berlin Wall. He *had* to interact with her because of his position. (Of course, he
didn't have to interact improperly.) Attractive women *will* pass through your mental
defense perimeter, but they must be allowed to enter only for appropriate reasons and
purposes, just as things are handled at any border crossing.

Manning the Customs Station

Once your perimeter goes up, what happens at your mental customs station? Say
your company hires a new coworker, Rachel. On her first day, Rachel walks around
the corner, starts talking, and *wham!* You're attracted. From this point, either she
can be processed properly in your mind without generating impure thoughts, or you
can mishandle the situation.

What happens next is critical to the purity of your mind.

You continue interacting with Rachel over time. The early interactions feed the
attraction. For instance, Rachel might return your attraction signals. Or her sense
of humor may match yours. She loves your favorite pizza. She's simply mad about
football. Rachel is refreshing and fascinating, so you love to think about her.

At this point, improper processing can carry you away into sensual thoughts or
other impure practices, like flirting and teasing in spite of being married. At worst,
you can be swept away like the foolish young man in Proverbs 7:

With persuasive words she led him astray;
 she seduced him with her smooth talk.
All at once he followed her
 like an ox going to the slaughter,
like a deer stepping into a noose
 till an arrow pierces his liver,   .
like a bird darting into a snare,
 little knowing it will cost him his life. (verses 21–23)

Your mind gets lost in the attractions. It doesn't really matter that you don't know Rachel very well. Early in the relationship, the mind is nimble in filling in the blanks with its creative imagination. That's part of the fun. The less you know about her, the more blanks there are to fill, and the more your mind can run with its fanciful thoughts. With further interaction, however, more facts dribble in. With fewer blanks to fill, the mind quickly gets bored. Facts are the killer virus of attractions.

What kind of facts? Once you've heard her talk about her wonderful new baby and how great her husband is, it becomes harder to imagine Rachel as your enchantress in waiting. She falls off your attraction screen and becomes merely a friend or coworker.

From Fred: Learning the Right Mental Processing

We get used to this kind of improper processing from our earliest days. Probably all of us can think of an example from high school where our minds got lost in our attractions. I had one in high school; her name was Judy.

I noticed her early in my senior year, when Judy was a junior. You talk about hitting attraction buttons! I was carried away into a land of silly dreaminess whenever I thought about her. I thought about what I would say and how we would love each other and where we would go, my mind filling in thousands of blanks, since I knew nothing about Judy except her name and her grade.

All year long I pined for her, watching her bounce merrily by, yearning for the day we could finally speak. I ached to ask her for a date, but I lacked courage. Even though I was the superstud athlete of the year, my heart turned to raspberry Jell-O when it came to girls.

As the year wound down, one chance remained: the senior prom. Struggling fiercely with my fears, I dialed her phone number. After some meaningless small talk, I stammered out my request. She actually said yes! Her melodious voice affirmed my existence, and you can imagine what my mind did with that.

I found the perfect place to take her after the prom dance: the Ironmen Inn. While the traditional site for after-prom dinners was the Highlander, I decided that I couldn't give my newfound love something so trite and dreary. In the secluded, curtained booths at the Ironmen, we could sit transfixed and not be interrupted on that glorious first night of the rest of our lives together.

After being escorted to our romantic private booth, we bantered lightly, my heart pounding deeply within me. My attraction grew with each passing moment. Judy's ravishing face glowed, and her lovely, full lips parted to speak. Enchanted, I listened dreamily, only to hear her say, "You know, I don't know how to say this, but I really, really wanted to go to the Highlander. Do you mind if we go over there?"

Clunk.

Although my attraction for her shuddered wildly, chivalry and honor carried the day. Mustering an air of nonchalance, I responded, "Sure, I guess not," though I knew this wasn't good for our date.

We had no reservations at the Highlander, of course. As we stood waiting to be seated, Judy brazenly asked, "Do you mind if I go over to Joel's table for a while?" She left me and spent the rest of the night with Joel and his date.

After finally being seated, I ate alone with my thoughts, musing, *This is why I like football better than girls.*

Later, Judy graciously threw me a bone, allowing me the honor of driving Her Highness home. On the way, she confided that she'd hoped all along to find a way to be with Joel that night since he hadn't asked her to the prom as she had expected.

Ugh.

My attractions to Judy died that night. The ugly facts—the killer virus of attractions—did them in! Initially, I didn't process my attractions to her properly, using emotional fantasy to fill in the blanks wherever I had no actual knowledge of who she was.

But let me share an example of someone who *did* process attractions well. Carter told me about Emma, a new woman in his engineering department. When he first saw her, she was giving a presentation to the whole group, and he was hit between the eyes:

"I was sitting there expecting another boring presentation when up bops Emma. She was pretty and intelligent, yet she had an airy disposition. She reminded me so much of the girls I knew back in college. My mind kept insisting, *I've got to get to know this girl.* But I was married, and I knew I shouldn't.

"My mind kept demanding to think about her. She seemed so attractive, but I knew I shouldn't think about her. Over the next few weeks, I purposely spent very little time around her and didn't talk to her unless I absolutely had to. I kept starving my eyes of her as well.

"Then I found out she'd just had a baby, and all she could do was talk about her new daughter. She plainly loved her husband very much. At this time, my attractions went down but not quite out.

"Later, some of the new engineering processes she put into place began to take some heavy criticism, and I saw that Emma's disposition wasn't so light and airy after all. She could be downright shrewish! Today, she's just a friend. I'm not even attracted to her anymore."

Starving the Attractions

That was proper processing. Emma had an entry visa into Carter's life because they worked at the same place, but the attractions were processed properly and generated few impure thoughts. That's what a good mental customs station does for you. We can't eliminate attractive women from our lives, but we can shield ourselves from the early attraction phase until they become only friends. Let's call this proper processing starving the attractions.

It's a concept that reminds me of an old cheer from my college days at Stanford:

If you can't win, cheat!

If you can't cheat, stall!

If you can't stall, quit!

Less than admirable, but funny in its way and somewhat applicable here. Starving the attractions is a stall tactic. Active stalling waits for the facts that will quickly process the relationship beyond the danger zone, where it generates no impurity.

What happens if we don't starve the attractions? What if we play with the attractions a little? Won't the passage of time kill the attractions anyway?

Most of the time, yes, but why take that chance? An improper relationship is not pleasing to God no matter how innocent it appears, and it threatens everything you hold dear in life at home.

In summary, you have a mind that runs where it wills. It must be tamed. Your best tactic is to starve the attractions, limiting the generation of impure thoughts and the damage they bring to your marriage relationship.

A Corral for Your Mustang Mind

As we said earlier, our minds are like wild mustangs running free. Mustangs have two characteristics in common with the male brain. First, the mustang runs where he wills. Second, the mustang mates where he wills and with whom he chooses, and there are mares everywhere! And if the mustang doesn't happen to see one nearby, he'll sniff the wind and, sensing the mare over the horizon, trot over the hill to mate.

This trait is similar to the wild donkey that God talked about through the prophet Jeremiah:

A wild donkey accustomed to the desert,
    sniffing the wind in her craving—
    in her heat who can restrain her?
Any males that pursue her need not tire themselves;
    at mating time they will find her. (Jeremiah 2:24)

Can you control the mustang? Can you run him down on foot or simply wag your finger and admonish him? No, of course not. Then how do you keep him from running and mating where he wills?

With a corral.

Currently, your mind runs like a mustang. What's more, your mind "mates" where it wills with attractive, sensual women. They're everywhere. With a mustang mind, how do you stop the running and the mating? With a corral around your mind.

Let's expand a bit on this metaphor to help you better understand our goal of reining in our roving minds.

Once, you were a proud mustang, wild and free. Sleek and rippling, you ranged the hills and valleys, running and mating, the master of your destiny. God, owner of a large local ranch, noticed you from a distance as He worked His herd. Though you took no notice of Him, He loved you and desired to make you His own. He sought after you in many ways, but you darted away from Him again and again.

One day He found you trapped in a deep, dark canyon with no way out. With the lariat of salvation, He gently drew you near, and you became one of His own. He desired to break you, that you might be useful to Him and bring Him further joy. But knowing your natural ways and how you loved to run free with the mares, He set a fence around you. This corral was the perimeter of the eyes. It stopped the running and kept you from sniffing the winds and running wildly over the horizon.

But while the corral stopped the *running*, it hadn't yet stopped the *mating*. You mated in your mind, through your attractions, thoughts, and fantasy, flirting and neighing lustily at the mares inside or near your corral. You had to be broken.

Closer and Closer

To help break you and your bad habits, let's take a look at four common categories of attractions that regularly come a married guy's way. How might you process these situations properly?

The first category is your visual attraction to the strangers we spoke of earlier: the joggers, receptionists, and online beauties. Because we've established a defense perimeter of the eyes—our corral—these are now over the horizon. We can't run there anymore. They no longer create attractions.

But there are still plenty of attractions within range of the corral. Categories two through four include the women who are not strangers, the women you interact with in life—the live attractions.

In category two are the women who aren't attractive to you and don't generate impure thoughts. They can include your friends, acquaintances, coworkers, and church members.

Your friend Dylan may notice someone and say, "Wow, look at her! She's hot!" You respond in mild surprise, saying, "I guess so. I've worked with her so long that I don't even think of her in those terms. She's just a friend."

Your defense against this category of women is a simple monitoring to make sure you notice early if one of them takes a step toward your corral.

The third category is likely the most dangerous of all. These are the women you know and interact with and who hit your attractions buttons, like Rachel, your new coworker, or maybe the new worship leader who thrills your soul with her worshipful heart. You neigh, drawing her toward your corral, if only in your mind.

Perhaps one of them has noticed you as well. Attracted to you, she trots purposefully toward your corral. Flattered, you snort majestically and stomp your foot and toss your head. Looking at her brings much pleasure. Pushing the boundaries, you stretch your head over the fence, nuzzling a bit through private lunches and close conversations. Worst of all, your mustang mind can do something a real mustang could never do: open the gate of the corral, and not just mentally.

Mason told us of a cousin who divorced his wife of twenty-six years after falling head over heels for another woman. "I just didn't know what to say to my cousin," he told us. "He got carried away, and he wasn't going to stop seeing her. There was just no talking to him."

You might say you could never open the gate of your corral to someone in the way Mason's cousin did. But look at statistics for the church—the divorce rates are way too high! Too many Christian couples are separating or recovering from adulterous affairs spawned by men who opened the corral of their minds. Without defenses, it could happen to you.

The last category includes those women who are already inside your mental corral. Your first thought may be that only your wife is in this category, but there are others God has placed close to you. This category can include the wife of your close friend. You'll share restaurant tables with them, create joyful memories with them, and pray earnestly with them. Emotionally, you'll be close. But you must not lurk.

Also inside your corral may be an old girlfriend to whom you're still deeply attached. She was in your corral long before your wife was, but you've never sent her out of your corral and back over the horizon. You mate easily with her in your mind because of your many trysts. Mentally, she's still right with you.

Then there might be an ex-wife, perhaps the mother of your children. Because of those precious little ones, she'll usually live near you. Because of your former intimacy, she may seem yours for the taking, in your mind. You remember the thrills, and you feel free to play with the thoughts. But you must lead her out of your corral and toward the safety of the horizon as well.

The perimeter of the mind processes the live attractions that canter up over the horizon and pass our corrals. By our starving the attractions, these women retreat to safety zones of friendship or acquaintance, where they no longer threaten our purity. Remember what Carter said about Emma? After he starved the attractions, she became "just a friend," and he wasn't attracted to her anymore.

Most women won't hit any attraction buttons at all, of course. As they enter your life, they simply trot past your corral toward the horizon again. You don't notice them, and they don't notice you. They are and will be merely friends, acquaintances, and coworkers, cavorting about on the horizon. But those who *do* attract you and *do* approach your corral must not be given any reason to come closer or to even approach the gate, where you just might, in a moment of weakness, let them in.

Preventing Sad Stories

Don't you owe it to your wife to put up a mental defense perimeter? You must protect your wife and kids from attractions outside your corral; otherwise, you'll have a sad story to tell, like the one we heard from Jake.

Jake was involved in full-time Christian ministry, standing strong. He had no mental defense perimeter, however, because he blissfully thought he didn't need one. As a result, he was unprepared when someone approached his corral. He told us, "Emily attended my church and was involved in the music ministry. Because of my skills and position in the church, I was involved in many activities with her. We were in a small worship band, and during practices, I noticed she began smiling in that certain way. She was pretty and I was attracted, but I didn't give it much thought until she kept on smiling at me. I got to thinking about it. The attractions were growing, and I felt a little excited and pleased with myself.

"One day, she stopped by my office and caught me alone. She began pouring out her troubles she was having with her husband. As a minister, I often did counseling, so I felt I should listen. She started crying and I put my arms around her, feeling sorry for her. She snuggled in a little, and I kind of liked it. She left, and nothing came of it, but now I was thinking about her constantly.

"Emily and I happened to take the same road to work, and I noticed she would be watching for me each morning, waving and smiling if she saw me. At practice, she was more and more flattering of my musical talents. She looked at me with those eyes even when I preached, smiling slightly though sitting right next to her husband. It was kind of naughty and thrilling.

"I began doing the strangest things, like driving miles out of my way to drive by her office just to see her car. What in the world did I gain by seeing her car, for Pete's sake? But it was romantic somehow. Finally, a few weeks later we were alone, and I kissed her. I knew that kiss would end my career at my church, but I couldn't help myself. The attraction had grown too strong."

Jake's career, marriage, and relationships with his children were severely damaged that afternoon. He once believed it could never happen, but it did happen because he lacked a defense perimeter and a proper mental customs station.

Friend, your wife and kids deserve a defense. You never know who will gallop near your corral.

15

Approaching Your Corral

L et's discuss another helpful way of categorizing the live attractions in a married guy's life that you must process safely across your borders.

There are two types of women who will approach your corral:

- Women who you find attractive
- Women who find you attractive

Both categories require similar defenses, and each is designed to starve the attractions until the women trot off toward the horizon again. Here's a closer look.

Women Who You Find Attractive

If you find someone attractive, your first line of defense is to take on the proper mind-set, which is, *This attraction threatens everything I hold dear.*

It may not appear threatening early in the attraction, when everything seems innocent. Remember, though, that attractions grow quickly and can destroy your marriage. But even if your marriage is never really threatened, the lurking will still weaken the foundation of your marriage and rob your wife of your full captivation. God hates that for His daughter.

Your second line of defense is to declare, *I have no right to think these things.* State this to yourself plainly, decisively, and often. Transform your brain to understand your rights, because your rights are clear here: you have none. *Who are you to be at-tracted to her? Didn't your Master already give you your wife? Doesn't He own you outright, at a steep price?*

The third line of defense is to heighten your alert. What do you normally do when you feel physically threatened? You take off your jacket and breathe deeply. You ready yourself for what's coming.

Suppose you are working security at a small concert venue, checking IDs and tickets, joking with the customers. One night, three men in black leather loudly roar up on motorcycles, looking surly and arrogant. Would you relax and back away from the door and keep joking around? Not on your life. Without hesitation, you'd step up to the door and stand erect, ready to confront the potential threat.

Consider the many *Star Trek* television series and movies. What did each star-ship captain cry when danger approached? "Red alert! Shields up!" In a similar vein, when an attractive woman approaches your corral, your defense perimeter must im-mediately respond, *Red alert! Shields up!*

With your mind-set transformed, you won't let her near the corral. The attrac-tion will begin to starve immediately, and she'll drift back toward the horizon.

How can you make sure that will happen?

Bounce your eyes. You saw her passing your corral, and you were physically attracted to her. Starve this attraction by bouncing your eyes. Don't dwell on her beauty by stealing glances. Bounce your eyes with zeal.

Avoid her. Sometimes this isn't possible, but do it when you can. If she works with you, and the two of you are assigned to the same project, don't ask her to eat lunch with you or offer her a ride home. Until the attraction phase dies, avoid op-portunities that create positive experiences with her. If she asks you to do something with her, excuse yourself.

Play the dweeb. When you're in her company, play the dweeb. Meet your new hero in our battle: Dweebman. He steps into a nearby public restroom and emerges as the polyester-clad enemy of all things flirtatious and hip. Dull, mild-mannered Dweebman—pocket protector shielding his heart and hair slightly askew—wages his quiet, thankless war of boring interchange. Our once-threatening Wondrous Woman withdraws to undefended sectors, leaving Dweebman victorious again in his never-ending good fight to stave off the hip and the impure in his galactic empire!

Okay, there's not *that* much glory in playing the dweeb. There'll be no comic book deals, no endorsements, no cable news interviews, but you'll be a hero to your wife and kids.

A dweeb is the opposite of a player. In relationships, players send and receive social signals smoothly. Dweebs do not. When a player wants to send attraction signals, there are certain things he'll do. He'll flirt. He'll banter. He'll smile with a knowing look. He'll talk about hip things. In short, he'll be cool. You were a player at one time. You knew how to feed attractions. You spent your whole adolescence learning how to do it.

As a married man, however, a little social suicide is very much in order. Always play the dweeb. Players flirt; learn to unflirt. Players banter; learn to unbanter. If a woman smiles with a knowing look, learn to smile with a slightly confused look, to unsmile. If she talks about things that are hip, talk about things that are unhip to her, like your wife and kids. She'll find you pleasant enough but rather bland and uninteresting. *Perfect.*

Sometimes a woman's attractiveness to you will be mental rather than physical. This is common in work environments as you work with women on projects that interest you both. In business, it's common to spend more hours per day with female coworkers than with your wife. You talk with them about common goals and achieving success, while all you and your wife talk about are the kids' discipline problems, who's going to change the dirty diapers, and bills, bills, bills.

In the same way as when you're around physically attractive women, you must understand that if your shields aren't up and you don't recognize the threat to your marriage, you're flirting with danger in any relationship that could blossom mentally or emotionally.

To summarize: If you're attracted to a woman, it doesn't mean you may never again have any sort of relationship or friendship with her. It only means you must up your defense perimeters. Once you've starved the attractions and she's a safe distance away, you can have a proper relationship, one that is honoring to your wife and to the Lord.

Women Who Find You Attractive

No matter our age (or our waistlines), we're still capable of thinking preposterous things like, *Finally, here is a woman who clearly has good taste and knows "handsome" when she sees it. I simply must get to know her better.* Yes, guys still make those statements.

Lucas, being short on cash, took a second job working an early shift at FedEx to make ends meet. He was simply doing what a man should do for his family during a serious financial crunch. Then Christi, an aggressive, attractive dispatcher, pranced by Lucas's corral and said, "You're so cute and sexy! I love to wrap my legs around men like you!" She bantered and flirted at every turn, teasing with double entendres and come-ons. She spread her legs slightly whenever they talked, and her shirt often flopped open for him.

One day she said, "My husband is out of town hunting for the weekend. I'm going to be so lonely." *Red alert! Shields up!* An hour later, Lucas found her house key on his desk with a note saying, "I've left you this key in case you need to get into my house this weekend!"

Lucas, to his credit, returned her key and let it be known in no uncertain terms that he would not be coming, and he asked her to stop what she was doing. Lucas kept the gate to his corral closed because Christi was threatening everything he held dear.

These days, Lucas could go to Human Resources and report that Christi was sexually harassing him, but getting into a "she said, he said" with a female manager could also be problematic. Today's supercharged "sexual harassment" environment is just one more great reason for a good defense perimeter. One wrong aside, one wrong suggestive comment, and you could land in huge trouble—and it could cost you your career.

It's all about awareness of your surroundings. If a gang of roving teens was outside your home, approaching with knives and baseball bats, you would sense a threat. *Red alert! Shields up!* Just as dangerous is the woman who finds you attractive. You must stop her by not returning any attraction signals. If she's a non-Christian, she's even more dangerous since she has no moral reason not to go to bed with you. Your second line of defense is using your shield of rights: *I have no right to think these thoughts, and I have no right to return these signals!* Jesus died a bloody death on the cross to purchase you. He has all the rights here. You have none. Speak this out loud to yourself again and again to rein in the mustang mind.

Don't dawdle about getting your shields up either. In one *Star Trek* movie plot, the enemy had captured a Federation starship and was approaching Captain Kirk and the USS *Enterprise* (the good guys). The enemy commander didn't respond to any calls as Kirk hailed him repeatedly. The enemy commander simply sneered, "Let them eat static."

Kirk found this lack of response peculiar. Confused and unsure of the intentions of the approaching ship, he dawdled. He did not put up his shields. Finally, when close enough, the enemy blasted away, severely disabling the *Enterprise*. In the very same way, you don't know what a woman's intentions are when she approaches your corral. Maybe you're misreading her bright, outgoing personality and she isn't attracted to you at all. Maybe she greets everyone that way. Maybe not. There may be an enemy on that ship. Maybe not. Just get your shields up and ask questions later. So what do you do when someone finds you attractive? How do you starve *these* attractions? Here are some guidelines:

- *Avoid her.* Spend absolutely no time alone with this woman, even in public places. The reason is simple: you don't want to feed her attractions. Make it obvious you aren't returning her interest.
- *Flee from her.* Don't smile knowingly at her. Don't join her prayer group. Don't join her worship team. Avoid working with her on a committee. Don't be anywhere that she can be further impressed with you. Do this consciously and methodically.
- *Prepare with "war-game" simulations.* What will you say if she calls you at work? What will you do if she invites you to lunch? Author Josh McDowell tells teens to decide what they'll do in the back seat of the car before they ever get to the back seat of the car. Otherwise, passion rules and your reasoning isn't clear. As adults, we applaud his advice to teenagers. Why not follow Josh's words ourselves?
- *Send absolutely no return attraction signals.* Don't answer the call. Let her "eat static"!

- *Help her out by playing the dweeb.* Show her that her initial attraction to you was a ridiculous mistake. Choose to be boring, and do it faithfully and fastidiously. Later, when she's no longer attracted to you, you can be your normal, interesting self again.

From Steve: Beware of Fascination Gratification

There is one more bit of enemy treachery that I want to address. In the counseling arena, we call it fascination gratification, and you need to recognize it now so that it can never sneak up on you. There is a dangerous place where you may have complete control of your lusty eyes and where pornography has been put soundly in its place and yet you're still sliding over the thinnest of ice in your relationships with women.

If it sounds hard to imagine, let me paint a quick word picture for you. Shortly after *Every Man's Battle* was published, a world-famous minister was caught alone with a young woman from his church, sitting beside a lake talking. He claimed the relationship was innocent and completely platonic. After a thorough investigation, it was determined that this pastor had never touched this woman or any of the other "lakeside women" who came forward to share their own stories about hanging out on the shoreline with their pastor.

So, were these relationships platonic, just as he'd claimed? Definitely, as they were not about *sexual* gratification. Were they innocent? Not so much, as they involved *fascination gratification.*

This man's marriage was dead and had been for some time. His mind was spinning in a dreadful depression, and his heart was barren and empty. Because of his position, he never considered altering his dark moods through drink or drugs, but he happily stumbled upon something else that did the trick: being in the presence of a woman who found him to be, well, fascinating. As he talked and shared his deep wisdom with her, he loved watching her listen in awe.

He found that preaching to thousands left him drained but that preaching to one awestruck heart energized him and that the gratifying, undivided, idealized attention of an adoring, attractive woman filled his sails.

You may never sink to such extremes, but that's not the point. Be vigilant when drawing deep gratification and satisfaction from adoring, platonic eyes around your corral. If you find you're intentionally saying things to bring greater attention to yourself and are using women to alter your moods, it could genuinely be considered acting out.

So, if your marriage is dead, we say resurrect it. That is God's will for you—there can be no mistake about that. Fight for it. Find out why things died and change those things.

Take your *wife* to the shoreline to talk. Teach *her* heart and eyes to adore you again. Don't draw from your "innocent" counterfeits, and don't stop pursuing your wife at any false finish lines. Be authentic. Your marriage is your great adventure, so live it out like a man. Be energized as you defend your home and fill your sails there.

If you're concerned that you might not spot the trickier mistakes that you might trip into with the opposite sex (like fascination gratification), let me present you with a simple filter of behavior that will protect your marriage and allow your relationship to thrive. While it won't solve *every* problem, it'll be helpful in dispersing confusion and evaluating right from wrong.

When it comes to your own sexual behavior:

1. It must be known by your wife.
2. It must be approved by your wife.
3. It must always involve your wife.

When it comes to any general, daily interaction with a woman:

1. It must be known by your wife.
2. It must be approved by your wife.

If you're doing something that does not meet these standards, whether sexual or nonsexual, then you are likely doing something that is not honoring God, your marriage, your wife, or yourself. You are also doing something that can be changed, if you are willing.

16

Inside Your Corral

For those women who are already within your corral, the situation can become rather complicated. These women won't naturally drift back to the horizon once the attractions dissipate. They're in your corral today and probably will be there tomorrow and the next day. This means you must eliminate these attractions in some other fashion.

Let's take a look at the two main categories of women within your corral:

- Old girlfriends and ex-wives
- Wives of your friends

Again, not every woman in these categories will be attractive to you. But if one of these women catches your fancy or has retained a piece of your heart, something must be done proactively. Each category has unique dangers, and each demands unique defenses, so let's take a look at what we should do.

From Fred: Old Flame

An old girlfriend or an ex-wife can be deadly to mental purity. Such attractions break you down in two ways:

- They weaken your ability to move toward one flesh with your wife.
- They enable Satan to fire a cruise missile, with little warning, into your marriage.

I had a heart-stopping summer romance with Abby following my freshman year of college. At the end of the summer, I left her to return to school in California. Lonely and heartsick, I wandered aimlessly through my days, feeling sorry for myself. We wrote every day and telephoned often. This went on for much of the fall quarter.

One day during an intramural football game, my eyes caught sight of a female referee. She looked like a grown-up version of my childhood sweetheart, Melody, who had moved to Canada when we were in the third grade.

After the game, I walked up and asked her what her name was (that was the extent of my "lines" in those days). Had she said, "Melody," I'd have instantly fallen for her. Instead, she said her name was Betsy, and I fell for her instantly anyway. (As you can see, if anyone ever needed good defenses, it was me!)

Meanwhile, Abby wondered why the letters and phone calls had dwindled. When I finally got the nerve to tell her there was someone else in my life, she was hurt deeply. When my little relationship with Betsy ended, I asked Abby for mercy and a second chance, but she would have none of it. Loyalty meant everything to her, and my breach of loyalty killed any attraction she felt for me.

But I was no quitter. I fought on, longing for her for many years. Whenever I had a new girlfriend and things turned stormy, I dreamed of Abby, wishing she were mine. "Everything would be different with Abby," I'd moan.

Abby eventually married and had a child. But I was still so hooked that after she separated from her husband for a time, I begged for her love again. (This was before I met Brenda, of course.) "Kids, debts, baggage—I'll carry them all, just to have you back," I begged. You could have made a syrupy movie about my addiction to Abby.

It's no wonder that when I finally fell in love with Brenda and married her, I expected our marriage to match up to this image of undying love I'd created around Abby. But I didn't know what was coming. A tranquil tunnel of love? More like a roller coaster!

Brenda and I have had our share of fights, the first starting on our wedding night. In fact, at times during our first two tumultuous years of marriage, I wished I had never heard of the institution. Most of our conflicts were over in-laws, especially after my family engaged my bride in an all-out war and I got caught in the cross fire.

The fights were hot and withering. Being young, we didn't yet know how to fight fair with each other or with our family members, so the collateral damage was great; Brenda and I each suffered major losses.

Guess who popped into my thought life? As my marriage spiraled downward, Abby spiraled upward into my thoughts. *Well, Abby always got along with my family. They loved her.* Around the holidays, I mused how peaceful life would have been with Abby instead. *Why can't Brenda get along with my family? After all, Abby could!*

No Right

One night I was driving toward home on an Iowa road between Fort Dodge and Harcourt. The moon was full, the air crisp and clear. As Abby popped into my head, an insight from God popped in as well. *You have no right to any relationship of any sort with Abby anymore, not even in your thoughts.*

"What?" I whined. "Lord, no right to even think about her?"

That's right, buddy. No right to even think of her.

How stark! My mind rebelled fiercely against Him, and the fight was on. My mind *liked* Abby, and it fought for her. In the end, however, truth prevailed.

It was inevitable. Maybe you already know from personal experience that God is a really tough and superior wrestler. Before we'd grappled together for even a few minutes, I was pinned flat and ready to agree with Him and stand on His side of the issue. What had seemed so unfair only moments earlier now seemed self-evident. I knew I'd forsaken all others on my wedding day. Now that promise had to become true in practice, not just in words.

Abby had been a girlfriend and had long been inside my corral, but it was time for me to open the gate and show her out. She had a husband whose hopes and dreams were tied up in her, and she had children who loved her. I had no right to my thoughts, even if Abby knew nothing of them (and she didn't). Besides, Brenda deserved better from me. I was her husband. Her protector.

First, I obliterated all memory anchors, destroying every old card, letter, and picture of her. All physical traces of Abby were eliminated from my world, just as God's people were supposed to do with the Canaanites when they entered the Promised Land.

These actions improved the situation, but Abby's anchors weren't the only issue here. I had to destroy my memories of her as well because they stood in opposition to God's desires and hopes for my marriage. I had often used these memories to salve my emotional pain. Now I had to lose the synaptic pathways that I'd built up around them.

How will I do that? I wondered. I wasn't sure, but I had to try.

First, I prayed for understanding and insight since I didn't know what I was doing. Then I stumbled ahead as best I knew how. I began by using the shield of rights every time Abby entered my head. I coldly stated, *I have no right to think about Abby, and I won't.*

Having said that, I would sing a hymn. Why? In the early days, I found that I couldn't quite capture a thought of Abby and just toss it, even though that is exactly what the Word commanded me to do. I soon realized that while I couldn't directly *capture* the thought, I could *replace* it with something else. That's why I would sing a hymn, out loud if I was alone or in my mind if I was in public. Once I began singing, the lyrics of the hymn replaced my thoughts of Abby.

Sometimes "Abby thoughts" rushed back in at the end of the hymn, so I'd start singing a second song. Abby might immediately return after that one too, so sometimes it took numerous hymns to send those thoughts packing. In due time, however, I'd always win the skirmish, but if the Abby thoughts returned in a few hours or days, I'd fight—and sing—again. To make sure I always had enough arrows in my quiver, at one time I had all four verses of more than fifty hymns memorized.

It was quite a war at first. During those days, I remember thinking, *I cannot take chances by simply detaining these captive thoughts in a detention center. I must nuke these thoughts!* While that was a bit corny, I knew there must be no question of victory when this battle was over.

Over time I began winning decisively, and an amazing thing happened without any personal effort. As I became proficient at the lesser level of control needed for *replacing* those thoughts of Abby, my mind naturally developed a higher level of control that's required for *capturing* those thoughts. Once that happened, I could actually grab an incoming impure Abby thought and toss it out of my head without singing. I could simply will it to be gone.

Eventually, something even more amazing transpired: my brain stopped bringing up thoughts of Abby altogether. As my custom station, my brain finally understood that Abby thoughts were unapproved and began policing those thoughts on its own at the subconscious level. Today, I don't think of Abby at all, no matter what my emotions or relational situations. The old mental pathways are now impassable.

Satan's Cruise Missiles

As mentioned earlier, however, there's a second danger in not taking care of business with the attractions inside the corral. If you're careless, Satan can fire a cruise missile into your marriage and shatter your world in a moment.

Years ago, I noticed a problem with Dan, a married friend. Several times when I was at his home, I noticed his finger hesitate on the TV remote when passing sex scenes on the movie channels. While the hesitation was nearly imperceptible, I saw it easily because of my own dark history. His eyes had no defenses, so I knew what he'd been watching when no one was around. What I didn't know, until it was too late, was what he'd also been *thinking*.

Dan and his wife were having problems. To him, the worst was the sexual frustration. "Joann just doesn't fulfill me," he told me. "It wouldn't take much because I don't ask for much. All I want is to French kiss with her. She just won't do it. We'll be messing around, and when things heat up, I'll try some French kissing. She always gets angry and pulls away. She says it's filthy and makes her nauseated. I don't see how French kissing is any filthier than any other kisses. It's the same saliva! Besides the Bible says that her body is not her own but actually mine. The Bible gives me the right to sexual fulfillment, and as my wife, she owes me sexual fulfillment in the way I want it. It isn't fair, and I don't know what to do."

This wasn't quite true, of course. In reality, Dan had already decided what to do. He turned his thoughts to his old girlfriend, a place where he could daydream about *her* French kisses and what might have been. She absolutely loved French kissing. Dan was ripe for the taking.

Of course, he didn't know that. After all, he hadn't heard from this old flame in years, and he figured his thoughts were harmless. What could they hurt? He didn't even know where she was these days, but Satan did. Out of the blue, she called Dan and said she'd be in town the following week. Dan's unguarded mind raced with the sensual possibilities at a time when his defense perimeters were already down.

The two of them landed in a hotel room. *Boom!* He didn't think it could happen to him, but in one smashing blow, his marriage was blasted to smithereens. He couldn't say no.

Bottom line: you have no right to any relationship with an old girlfriend or ex-wife if you still nurture an attraction to her.

Friends' Wives

You may think that affairs like Dan's happen so infrequently that you can confidently say, "Well, I would never do such a thing!" But words like that mean nothing if you have any sense. We urge you to please protect yourself. Don't be defenseless because you can get fooled.

Far too much is at stake to be sloppy with your defenses with anyone, and that includes the wives of your friends. If your best friend gave you all his worldly goods and told you to take care of them, you would probably invest wisely and take no chances, right? It's even more important that you take no chances with his wife, his most precious love of all.

Have you ever had an attraction to a friend's wife? Without defense perimeters, you've probably had many attractions like that. You're a man. Attractions happen. What do you do with those?

Again, you start with the truth: *I have no right to any relationship with my friend's wife apart from my relationship with my friend.* Remember especially that there's nothing more dangerous than talking to a friend's wife when things are dry in either your marriage or her marriage. It's not that you don't trust your friend's wife; it's that you don't want to start anything. She should be like a sister to you, with no hint of attraction between you.

You'll always have some relationship with your friend's wife, but limit it to when your friend is around. This isn't always possible, but these simple rules can shield you from surprise attacks within the corral:

1. Limit all conversations between you and your friend's spouse to when your wife or your friend is with you, especially if you are attracted to her. Keep things light and short.

2. If you happen to reach your friend's wife by call or text instead of your friend, get off with her promptly. Don't be rude, but keep your conversation with her brief. For any necessary texts with your friend's wife, such as working out logistics with the kids, create a group text that includes your spouse as well.

3. If you stop by your friend's house and he isn't home, she may invite you in. What do you do then? Politely decline to enter. What possible purpose is served by staying?

4. Capture any attractions toward your friend's wife and nuke them totally. Return to the rules of starving your eyes and taking such thoughts captive. Never, ever tell yourself, *Oh, I can handle it—no problem.* You need to deliberately tear away the thoughts so she doesn't see the attraction signals and decide to send back a few of her own. Leave her no opportunity to send a return signal.

You may view these precautions as overly rigid, but we're just counseling safety measures here. In practice day to day, this approach isn't restrictive because your friends' wives are with your friends most of the time anyway, so the rules don't apply that often. You're rarely alone with a friend's spouse.

Besides, all this is important to the Lord. What God has put together, let no man tear asunder. Protect your friend's hopes and dreams as diligently as you're protecting your own hopes and dreams. You're his friend. Given the number of divorces within the church, a simple defense perimeter is in order.

And some advice for a special situation: if you're single and a close female friend gets married, be willing to quickly and graciously let the friendship drift away. The reality is, marriage changes things. Though it's a somewhat mysterious truth, she's no longer the same person because she is now one flesh with another man. She needs to be about building her marital relationship and finding "couple friends" together with him.

From Fred: Learning a Lesson

Before I knew Brenda, my best friend was a woman named Hannah who lived in the apartment above me. She had a boyfriend to whom she was perfectly loyal, and I wasn't in the market for a girlfriend at the time, so we paired well. We would often sit for hours as she talked about her insecurities, fears, and frustrations. I had just moved back to Iowa from California, and she was my only close friend.

Then I met Brenda, whom I courted mostly by phone during our seven-month romance. Since she lived in a city three hours away, Brenda had little to do with Hannah. Shortly after we were married, I told Brenda that I was planning to have lunch with Hannah the following Wednesday.

"Why?" Brenda asked.

"To catch up on things, mostly."

"And I'm not invited?"

"Well, she's having some personal problems she wants to talk over with me, and since you don't know each other, she would probably feel uncomfortable sharing them in front of you."

"I'm not sure I like that."

"Why? We've always been just friends."

"Well, for one thing," she explained, "I'm not sure I'm comfortable with us having friends of the opposite sex without each other present. Besides, it looks bad for you to have lunch with a single woman alone. What if someone from church saw you? I just don't feel right about it."

"You trust me, don't you?"

"I trust you. And she has a boyfriend, so I trust her motives for now. But what if her motives change down the line? I won't be there to spot it."

I pondered Brenda's reasoning and eventually canceled the lunch date. I had to admit that she made sense, and as simple as that, I'd learned that it wasn't appropriate for me to have lunch alone with Hannah.

I was glad I listened to Brenda's advice. As my own marriage struggled during the first two years, I was glad I had to deal with only the memories of Abby. Had Hannah also been around, who knows what would have happened? Though we were never romantically involved, our close friendship might have turned romantic in the midst of my emotional crucible. As a new Christian, would I have been able to resist falling for her? Given my track record, I'm glad Brenda urged dismissal of that friendship early on.

Some would say that all such friendships with the opposite sex should die once one marries. While I wouldn't go that far, I will say that such friendships must be guarded. To be careful is to be wise. After all, your marriage is on the line.

Looking Ahead

Purifying your eyes and mind is more than a command—it's also a sacrifice. As you make that sacrifice, as you lay down your desires, your maturity in the Lord will grow and blessings will flow. Your spiritual life will experience new health, joy, and stability, and your marital life will blossom as you learn to sacrifice your own desires for hers.

Sacrificing your personal desires for the sake of your marriage and the kingdom lies at the core of your third defense perimeter, the one you must build around your heart. In fact, this final perimeter serves as the bedrock foundation for the first two perimeters of the eyes and mind. In other words, if this one fails, everything else will eventually fail in this battle too. Part 6 is all about the perimeter of the heart, so let's keep moving and learning how to live according to God's standards.

Part VI

Victory in Your Heart

17

Cherishing Your One and Only

Your outer defense perimeters—protecting your eyes and your mind—will defend against sexual sin and guarantee that your wife remains beyond compare in your eyes. This is absolutely crucial in reforming your brain's synaptic pathways to focus only on your wife and in finding long-term victory over sexual sin.

Perhaps you're wondering, *What exactly does long-term victory look like? What can I realistically expect if I implement these defenses?*

Well, when we say that these perimeters are absolutely crucial, we're not saying they work instantly, like waving a magic wand over your brain and penis. We've made it abundantly clear in this book that you can't expect full freedom by next Tuesday.

But we *can* say that, over time, for all practical purposes daily sexual temptation will literally dry up in your life. For instance, it has been well over twenty-five years since I (Fred) have masturbated. In fact, it has been over twenty-five years since I've even done a search of any kind for a sensual photo, clip, or movie on a television or computer for the purpose of lust.

It's not that I *can't* fall into sexual sin anymore. After all, I still have the same eyes with that same innate ability to run wild. It's just that I *don't*. I don't want to, and because God has given me everything I need to participate in the divine nature and to escape the corruption in my world caused by my own evil desires, I don't have to (see 2 Peter 1:3–4).

That is what we mean by long-term freedom. Yes, sexual sin is certainly every man's *battle,* but sexual freedom is every man's *destiny.* Will you rise up and walk in your destiny?

To help you achieve that destiny of freedom, let's now consider the third perimeter, that innermost perimeter of your heart. To build out this section of your defenses, you must be consumed with God's purposes to cherish your wife.

It may not immediately be clear how this inner perimeter—cherishing your wife with your heart—works to defend your purity, but it would be difficult to overstate its importance. In fact, the inner perimeter of the heart is the foundational bedrock upon which you build the superstructure of the two outer perimeters. If this inner foundation crumbles and gives way, the two outer perimeters will often crumble over time as well. Long-term freedom will never materialize.

Where Your Commitment to God Shows First

Let's take a deeper look at God's purposes in this regard. If Christians were consumed by God's purposes, it would first be reflected in our marriages. But the rates of divorce, adultery, and marital dissatisfaction in the church reveal the true state of our hearts.

We've known very few men consumed by their marriages and fewer still consumed by purity, yet God expects you to be consumed by both. God's purpose for marriage is that it parallel Christ's intimate, sacrificial relationship with His church so that you might be one with your wife.

But how does matching Christ's relationship to His church help you build the inner perimeter and defend your sexual purity? The answer begins in your heart, where you may have selfish attitudes and expectations of your wife in marriage. When she doesn't meet these expectations, you become grumpy and frustrated and you pull away from her in your heart: *Well, if this is how she's going to be, why should I go through all the effort of being pure? She doesn't deserve it.*

So you retaliate by withdrawing your heart and pulling away from your responsibilities to love and cherish her. Since God's standard of cherishing *always* includes being sexually true to your wife, once your commitment to cherishing her weakens, even bit by bit, your will to maintain the outer defense perimeters of your eyes and mind erodes along with it.

To cherish her means to treat her with tenderness and hold her dear. We're sure you *want* to feel that selfless, romantic urge to do so, but perhaps you aren't feeling it and are finding it difficult to cherish your one and only these days. We've been there, so we understand. What do you do in this case? *You cherish her anyway.*

The biblical command to cherish carries such heavy ramifications for your sexual purity and your marriage that you can't afford to leave it up to your feelings alone.

Christ's Example

For centuries, Solomon's Song of Songs has been viewed as an allegory of how Christ feels for His bride and how she feels in return. Keep that interpretation in mind as you read the following portions (condensed from Song of Songs chapters 4, 5, and 7). Look first at Jesus's feelings toward His bride:

> How beautiful you are, my darling!
>> Oh, how beautiful!
>> Your eyes behind your veil are doves. . . .
> Your lips are like a scarlet ribbon;
>> your mouth is lovely. . . .
> You are altogether beautiful, my darling;
>> there is no flaw in you. . . .
>
> You have stolen my heart, my sister, my bride;
>> you have stolen my heart
> with one glance of your eyes. . . .
> How delightful is your love, my sister, my bride! . . .
> Your head crowns you like Mount Carmel.
>> Your hair is like royal tapestry;
>> the king is held captive by its tresses.
> How beautiful you are and how pleasing,
>> my love, with your delights!
>> (4:1, 3, 7, 9–10; 7:5–6)

Now observe the church's feelings toward Jesus:

My beloved [husband] is radiant and ruddy,
    outstanding among ten thousand.
His head is purest gold;
    his hair is wavy
    and black as a raven. . . .
His mouth is sweetness itself;
    he is altogether lovely.
This is my beloved, this is my friend. . . .
I belong to my beloved,
    and his desire is for me. . . .
Let us go early to the vineyards . . .
    there I will give you my love.
The mandrakes send out their fragrance,
    and at our door is every delicacy,
both new and old,
    that I have stored up for you, my beloved.
    (5:10–11, 16; 7:10, 12–13)

Do you sense Jesus's desire for you as part of His bride? In return, does your heart yearn for Him like this?

Because our marriage relationships should parallel Christ's relationship to the church, our feelings for our wives should parallel these passages. Does your wife feel cherished like this?

These passages are a great reminder of how exciting marriage ought to be, especially when channeled toward the one God intended for you to have.

From Fred: Caught Up in Conditions

These excerpts from the Song of Songs by Solomon also serve as a great barometer to measure how you're handling God's purposes for your marriage. Are you sacrificially cherishing your wife? Do you feel those emotions for your wife as expressed in those passages? I will admit that I haven't always felt that way.

Do you remember pop quizzes from school, a sort of diabolical truth serum used by evil teachers to expose your knowledge (or lack of it) to the world? God loves pop quizzes, but He doesn't test our *knowledge* with them; He reveals our *character* and our *heart*.

God used pop quizzes a lot to expose my heart during our first two years of marriage when we were staggered by in-law problems with my family. Our marriage was quickly wilting away.

For example, one Valentine's Day I went to buy a card. Without warning, this turned into a pop quiz from God. Fingering through the cards, I read the texts. One by one I returned them to the rack as too mushy, too contrived, or too romantic. Little by little, panic settled in as I sensed the inevitable. Not one Valentine's card in the store could be sent by me with any measure of sincerity. The romance was gone, and my cherishing heart had withered to a dry husk.

Head down, I scurried from the store, recognizing the depth of our loss. My grade on the quiz? Sickening!

What about you? Has your heart for your wife withered?

If so, you probably got there the same way I did: by stopping short of God's purposes for marriage. God's primary standard is to unconditionally and sacrificially cherish her, no matter what. No conditions. But in America, we've mixed in our own ideas and diluted His standard, adding new, mealymouthed terms to create conditional contracts.

Take my case, for example. If I'd been living according to God's standards and purposes, I'd have added no conditions to my relationship with Brenda. But I did mix in a few. In my marriage, my conditions were that I would cherish Brenda *only* if she made peace with my family and shaped up in her attitude toward my leadership.

Whenever we set conditions like these, we fix our gazes on what we expect to get from the marriage for ourselves as the primary focus. Of course, matrimony *should* deliver more to each spouse than the single life does. In fact, in the premarriage classes I teach, I always ask, "What do you expect to get out of marriage that you can't get by staying single?" The answers are part of our bright hope for marriage.

Look at it this way: Husbands and wives both have needs and responsibilities in marriage. That's normal and expected. The trouble is, by nature we husbands tend to go about all this backward. We tend to focus upon *our* needs and *her* responsibilities to meet those needs.

But that's not how Jesus related to His bride. If you want to match up with His methods and build a strong inner defense perimeter around your heart, you must instead focus on *her* needs and *your* responsibilities to her. Laying your life down for your wife brings out the best in you and allows her to fully blossom under your leadership. But when you do it backward, you're expecting your wife to fulfill *your* needs and *your* dreams under some contractual conditions you've composed and laid heavily across her shoulders. In my case, anger and resentment erupted whenever I felt Brenda wasn't holding up her side of the bargain. She didn't meet the conditions, so I no longer felt like cherishing her.

With that kind of selfish and conditional focus, oneness in a marriage can't grow. For instance, Hunter said this about his wife:

> She was showing such a lack of ambition. What I expected when we got married was that we would both continue in our careers and really build our lives financially in those early years. She just wasn't doing what I thought she'd do, and she really seemed kind of lazy and selfish. Then she got pregnant, and after a few months she said, "I don't like the way I look anymore, so I don't want to have sex until after the baby comes." I found that brutal and so unfair.
>
> The more I thought about no sex, the more it bothered me, and I figured that if she were just going to live any way *she* pleased, then I would live any way *I* pleased. I had a biblical right to sexual fulfillment in marriage, and I was going to have it one way or another. That's how I came to have an affair.

Now that's a flimsy excuse for adultery, to be sure. But the important point to notice is that its seeds lay in Hunter's focus on what *he* was or was not getting out of the marriage.

These kinds of conditional contracts don't work, partly because they're written while you're dating, so they can't flex with life's circumstances. Regardless of how long you date or court her, you don't know each other well enough or the future well enough to craft a decent interpersonal contract that can cover the hidden or changing conditions of the heart, mind, and body as life happens.

For instance, how could I have anticipated the huge problems we'd have with my family as they attacked Brenda mercilessly? I'd never seen that side of my mom and my sisters, and I grew up with them! And how could Brenda have anticipated my out-of-control temper, which she'd never seen before our wedding night? As the months passed, she'd eventually see me punch holes in our walls with my bare fists and throw a pot of bean soup across the kitchen floor in rage. Neither of us expected this kind of chaos.

A conditional marriage contract originally defines what you hope to get out of marriage. But as time passes and you learn more about each other, and as life crashes in on you in a helter-skelter way, you add more expectations and more requirements of each other until you can hardly recognize the original agreement. *Wait a minute! This isn't working out like I expected. I'm getting out!*

Brenda and I came to just such a moment of truth sometime after I tossed that pot of bean soup. One morning, she sat down at the kitchen table across from me, looked me in the eye, and simply said, "I don't know how else to say this, so I'm just going to tell it to you straight. My feelings for you are dead." She wondered if we should consider divorce.

Hearing the word *divorce* dazed and shocked me. As a child of divorce, the old feelings of horror swept over me again. When my mom first told me she was divorcing dad, my heart raced with fear. *What are we going to do?* Terror now bolted through my heart again. *What am I going to do?*

No Matter How Much Gravel

Several days passed, with my mind disoriented in pain and confusion. One day when Brenda was at work, I opened my refrigerator and reached in for a half gallon of milk. Her words lay heavily upon my chest. I poured the milk, shut the refrigerator door, and paused. Tears flooded my eyes.

I had to make a stand.

Raising my right hand and pointing a finger toward heaven, I declared, "God, I don't care how much gravel I have to eat, I'll never get a divorce."

I finally understood the promise I'd made on my wedding day. My promise wasn't conditional. If she fed me meat and potatoes, I would eat it. If she fed me gravel, I would eat it. I was going to change or tolerate or love in whatever way necessary, but I would keep my promise to love and cherish her, whatever the cost, no matter what she did or didn't do.

"What does eating gravel have to do with cherishing?" you might ask. "Do I give up everything I have to keep peace? What about *my* rights?"

Well, you do have rights, and we're not saying your wife has no responsibility to cherish you in return. But in the countless ways we poke each other in this shared space called marriage, our focus needs to be on *our* sharp edges, not hers.

God always knew marriages would wither when rooted in conditional contracts, which is why He established an unconditional covenant instead. He knew that conditions can change.

You see, God never forgot what we often forget—namely, the curse of Eden is a grinding curse. Life is a steamroller, making pancakes of conditions and easily mashing the naive contracts we create for ourselves. In our dreams for marriage, maybe we forgot that we will still have to work long hours by the sweat of our brows to eat and to provide and that we won't always see each other as much as we wish. Maybe we forgot that we will sometimes be beaten up and used by bosses, our minds so numb that we just don't want to talk about what happened when we get home. Maybe we forgot that with the pain in childbirth comes bodies that may never regain their former shape.

Any number of trials and tribulations might make our pet conditions impossible to meet, but we press for them anyway, demanding some form of Eden from our marriages, when all the time our true responsibility is to cherish our wives sacrificially and unconditionally.

Trouble is, we don't like our place, and that kind of sacrifice doesn't sound much like Eden to us. So we let our inner defenses down, and we lose our concern for God's purposes for our marriage and, eventually, for our sexual purity. The defense perimeter around our heart is breached.

A Man with Complete Faithfulness

We now want to direct your attention to a man in the Bible who *did* like his place and who *did* love God's purposes. All men should be as faithful as he was, cherishing both their kings and their wives. This man's name was Uriah.

In 1 Chronicles 11:41, we see Uriah listed as one of David's "mighty warriors"— the men who "gave his kingship strong support to extend it over the whole land, as the LORD had promised" (verse 10).

Uriah was clearly consumed with the purposes of his king, David. He was also consumed with the purposes of God. Uriah was by David's side in the caves when Saul hounded their heels. He cried with David as their homes burned at Ziklag. He cheered himself hoarse at David's coronation, and he fearlessly fought to extend David's kingdom over the whole land. Swearing his life to the purposes of God, Uriah often stood in harm's way for David and his throne.

Sound familiar? You swore your life to someone in this way, didn't you? You swore before family and friends to honor and cherish your wife, abandoning all others. You promised she would have more from marriage than she had as a single girl, and you swore your life to the Lord's purposes, to sacrificially love her, come what may.

Are you consumed by this commitment? Consumed enough to live faithfully and to cherish her completely? Consumed enough to stand in harm's way and to eat gravel until God's purposes and your promises are finally established in your land?

Uriah was certainly that consumed. His faithfulness was complete, but alas, David's faithfulness was not. He went to bed with Bathsheba, Uriah's wife. When she became pregnant, David had a mess on his hands. As always, Uriah was out of town fighting David's battles. Bathsheba's pregnancy could mean only one thing: David—not Uriah—was the father.

David addressed the situation by fabricating a ruse. He ordered Uriah back from the front lines. David's plan was to quickly send Uriah home to a warm, cuddly night with Bathsheba. If David moved quickly enough, people would naturally assume the unborn child was Uriah's.

Tragically, Uriah's faithfulness to the king was so complete that David's plan didn't work:

David said to Uriah, "Go down to your house and wash your feet." So Uriah
left the palace, and a gift from the king was sent after him. But Uriah slept at
the entrance to the palace with all his master's servants and did not go down
to his house.

David was told, "Uriah did not go home." So he asked Uriah, "Haven't
you just come from a military campaign? Why didn't you go home?"

Uriah said to David, "The ark and Israel and Judah are staying in tents,
and my commander Joab and my lord's men are camped in the open country.
How could I go to my house to eat and drink and make love to my wife? As
surely as you live, I will not do such a thing!"

Then David said to him, "Stay here one more day, and tomorrow I will
send you back." So Uriah remained in Jerusalem that day and the next. At
David's invitation, he ate and drank with him, and David made him drunk.
But in the evening Uriah went out to sleep on his mat among his master's
servants; he did not go home. (2 Samuel 11:8–13)

Look at Uriah! He was so consumed by the purposes of God that he refused to
go to his house, even to wash his feet. His faithfulness was so strong that, even when
drunk, he didn't waver from his commitment and zeal. His purity of soul was so
great that no treacherous trick formed against him could stand. God wouldn't allow
David's simple deception to cover his immense sin against God and against God's
choice servant Uriah. God loved Uriah, and God loved Uriah's love for Bathsheba.

Uriah knew his place. He was satisfied to fill his role in God's purposes.

If we're to be like Uriah, we must know our place and be content with it.

Your Ewe Lamb

What does it mean to cherish? We needn't look further than Uriah's example.

After David arranged for Uriah to be killed in battle, God sent His prophet
Nathan to confront David about his sin. He used a word-picture story that revealed
Uriah's cherishing, loving heart toward Bathsheba:

The Lord sent Nathan to David. When he came to him, he said, "There were two men in a certain town, one rich and the other poor. The rich man had a very large number of sheep and cattle, but the poor man had nothing except one little ewe lamb he had bought. He raised it, and it grew up with him and his children. It shared his food, drank from his cup and even slept in his arms. It was like a daughter to him.

"Now a traveler came to the rich man, but the rich man refrained from taking one of his own sheep or cattle to prepare a meal for the traveler who had come to him. Instead, he took the ewe lamb that belonged to the poor man and prepared it for the one who had come to him." (2 Samuel 12:1–4)

The rich man in the story represented David, who saw Bathsheba only as someone he could devour to satisfy his sexual longings. But Uriah, "the poor man," saw his "lamb" as the joy of his life, his pet to cherish, to sleep in his arms. Uriah had only one wife; a faithful man like him could have only one. His ewe lamb, Bathsheba, bounced and pranced and frolicked and laughed with him, bringing him great joy.

The lamb "was like a daughter to him," the passage says. Do you have daughters? If so, you know what the Lord conveys here. A love for a daughter is special, and daughters are easy to cherish. When they smile, their eyes sparkle. We love to protect them and to tease them. We love to walk by the river, arm in arm, just to be with them. We love it most when they fall asleep in our arms. We cherish their very essence.

Is your wife *your* little ewe lamb?

You may feel uncomfortable with that imagery, and maybe it sounds chauvinistic to you. We're certainly not using it to describe relative levels of strength or ability. (From Fred: I know this from personal experience, as Brenda is an accomplished registered nurse and mother of four with firm views on everything. Yet in a tender moment when I told Brenda that I wanted to treat her like a "ewe lamb," she felt honored rather than offended.)

The Bible uses the term to capture a heavenly message. As Bathsheba was precious to Uriah, your wife is *your* precious one, your only one. She lives with you and lies in your arms. She's to be cherished, not because of what she does for you, but because of her essence, her value to God as a child born in His image. You've been entrusted with the priceless essence of another human soul, so precious to God that from the foundation of the world, He planned to pay His dearest price to buy her back again.

Regardless of the current rubble in your marriage or the list of unmet conditions, you owe God to cherish your wife's essence. When you look deeply enough into your wife's eyes, past the pain and hurts and fights, you can still find that little ewe lamb gazing back, hoping all things and trusting all things.

Whether You Feel It or Not

God entrusted your wife to you, and she placed herself in trust to you. How can we entrust such a valuable gift to a concept of cherishing based only on wispy feelings? Christians like to say, "Love is not a feeling; it's a commitment." Well, this is the time to heed those words. We owe that love always, despite our feelings.

In our society, we have sensitivity training and cultural-enrichment classes. We believe that if we can only teach people the "right" feelings, they'll act correctly. In the Bible, however, God tells us the opposite: we're first to act correctly, and then right feelings will follow.

If you don't feel like cherishing, cherish anyway. Your right feelings will arrive soon enough.

Remember, the Bible says that God loved us while we were yet sinners. Clearly, loving the unlovely is a foundation of God's character, and cherishing the unlovely is its bedrock. Since Christ died for the church—the unlovely—and since our marriages should parallel Christ's relationship to the church, we have no excuse when we don't cherish our wives. God loved us before we were worthy; we can do nothing less for our wives.

So let's move to the next chapter and explore what cherishing a wife looks like in practice.

18

Carrying the Honor

We've been talking about cherishing our wives and how we're to treat them with tenderness and to hold them dear, despite our feelings. Now we're going to consider what cherishing looks like in practice, day to day. As you read, let this chapter be a reminder to experience the wonder at what your wife's given you and the enormous honor it is to carry her baton.

Carry the honor nobly!

From Fred: Honor Both Her Heavenly and Earthly Father

As a father, I carry my daughter's baton. I was there when our first daughter, Laura, was born. I remember cradling her when she was sick as a toddler. Her fever was so high that her eyes rolled up into her head. After we rushed her to the doctor, she was so lethargic that she didn't even feel the shot that her pediatrician poked into her leg.

I remember the time she broke her finger when the car door slammed on it and I held her close. I remember the time she won a part in a play and I practiced with her again and again until she had her lines just right. I remember reviewing math flash cards with her until my eyes crossed, night after night.

When the volleyball was spiked at her feet three times in a row at the family reunion, I held her close so she could hide her tears in my chest as she sobbed, "They all think I'm no good." I stayed close to her for the rest of the day, defending her honor and brazenly daring another spike against my Peanut.

I labored over Laura's swimming strokes and sweated through my clothes when I taught her to ride her bike. I talked with her about middle school and how she was on the cusp of adolescence. I walked often to the altar with her, hand in hand, providing for her spiritual growth and understanding.

I learned to do her hair so she would always look nice, even when Mom was away. I bought her a few things she didn't really need—framed prints, cashew nuts—just because I knew she would love them.

I carry the baton of care for my daughter, and no hip haircut, fast car, or sweet smile will trick it out of my hand. My investment is too great. My son-in-law will owe me big, and he'd better honor her!

When I asked for Brenda's baton from my father-in-law, he was on his deathbed. He strengthened from time to time, but we both knew his time on earth was nearly over. I entered his hospital room much stronger than he but far more frightened. I knew how he loved his daughter. I knew how he once held her and let her cry when she came home with a squirrel-cut instead of a haircut. I knew how he proudly gave her a used red Chevy Nova as a gift. I knew how he used to swim way out into the ocean and let her sit on him like a raft, floating merrily. I knew how he had diligently raised her in purity, keeping her in church and away from ribald influences on her life.

I asked for her hand, and then he said something to me that has remained engraved indelibly in my memory over the years: "Though I don't know you well, I know you're the kind of man that will do what you say. I know you'll take care of her." Never in my life had a man believed in me so, trusting my manhood and entrusting me with something so valuable. He gave his only daughter, his cherished one, to me even while knowing he could never step back in to defend her if I didn't keep my word, that he would never be there to remind me of my promises, and that he would never be there to put that sparkle back in her eyes if I ever made it disappear.

I owe him because he trusted me. I owe him because he provided such a wonderful daughter to me. I owe him because of his great investment in her. When I see him again in heaven, I won't have to avert my eyes sheepishly in shame. He gave me the baton, and I will continue to run well with it.

I also owe her other Father. He saved my life from sin and picked me up from the ash heap and set me among princes. He adopted me and gave me the strength for today and a bright hope for tomorrow. And He saved a precious ewe lamb for me, a pure one without spot or blemish, with sparkling eyes and a soft heart. He formed her in the womb and looked on with joy when she crawled and then walked and talked. He saw her sing "Throw Out the Lifeline" before Him as a member of the Singing Cousins. He sent His only Son to provide for her future, to protect her, and to bring her home to heaven safely. God isn't amused when I neglect to nurture a cherishing heart for Brenda. He raised her and cherished her, so He thinks I must do the same.

With all my heart, I agree.

Remember What She Gives You

Your wife gave up her freedom for you. She relinquished her rights to seek happiness elsewhere. She exchanged this freedom for something she considered more valuable: your love and your word. Her dreams are tied up in you, dreams of sharing and communication and oneness.

She's pledged to be yours sexually. Her sexuality is her most guarded possession, her secret garden. She trusted you would be worthy of this gift, but you've regularly and cavalierly viewed sensual garbage, polluting and littering her garden. She deserves more, and you must honor that.

You must also cherish your wife because she shares her deepest secrets and longings with you. Brenda has told me stories she has told no one else. For instance, I know of a teasing word that, if I were to say it, would bring tears to her eyes instantly because of a trauma long ago. She's shared long-burning regrets and cried in my arms.

After years of marriage, I know what thrills her soul. I once entered a bookstore, leaving her waiting in the car. I purchased a book, passing over the good-customer limit to earn a five-dollar gift certificate. The cashier asked whether she should apply it to my current purchase, but I said, "No, I'll save it for my wife. She'll be real excited about it."

Just then, Brenda walked in. I whispered to the clerk, "Watch this!" I turned and gave the gift certificate to Brenda. She squealed out loud and, giggling, said, "Ooh, this is great!" The cashier laughed with me.

You see, I know Brenda. She is my beloved, and I am hers. I know her deepest fears, her desires for the future, and what she absolutely can and can't handle. She risked much in opening herself up so broadly to me, and I must have a cherishing heart in return, in honor of that risk.

When growing up, Brenda never feared anything because her dad was there. He never dishonored her, never shocked her, never frightened her or let her down. She traded all that for a guy with a short fuse who yelled and argued and called her names. I'm the one who upset her stomach, forcing her into unpleasant in-law situations without trying to understand, at times making her cower in tears. She never traded for that. She traded for a higher protection, but I gave her less.

Have you given less? Your wife risked much and traded much to marry you. Was it a good bargain for her?

Honor Her Hope

In my office, I keep an eight-by-ten black-and-white photo of Brenda from when she was a year old. Her little eyes sparkle and are filled with the hope and joy of life, her mischievous smile apparent even then with her glowing, chubby cheeks radiating joy and a carefree spirit. That face is so full of expectation and wonder. I brought that infant picture to my office because it reminds me that I need to honor that hope.

I'm a man, so through the years, I had a tendency to rebel. Life could get very hard sometimes, and work could drive me nearly out of my mind. I had four kids to provide for and a payroll to meet. I had church activities and sporting events and social obligations and on and on. Sometimes my heart began to crumble. At times, I could hear my rebellious side screaming for *my* rights and *my* way and *my* freedom. And sometimes I felt like jumping in the car and disappearing into the great northwest. Sad but true.

But I couldn't do it when I thought of Brenda. During long days of battle then and now, her baby picture always reminds me that she's my little ewe lamb, always hopeful, always believing in me, always looking ahead for "us." I want the sparkle of Brenda's baby eyes shining in her eyes today, decades later.

You must honor your wife with your own cherishing heart. God loved Uriah's love for Bathsheba. Does God love my love for Brenda? Does God love your love for your wife?

It doesn't matter what our wives look like, what they have or haven't done, or whether life has unfolded differently than we expected. We must honor and cherish them.

Clearly, life can unfold differently. Very differently. When Brenda and I first married, we were hoping to have four years together before having children, a time to build our relationship. We'd known each other only seven months on our wedding day. In addition, Brenda's dad had died two months before the wedding. She moved three hours away from her hometown to start our life together. She was aching over her father, and from that distance, she could not support her mother in her grief. We were searching for a church and had no friends. She had a new job and I was fairly new in mine. With me in commission sales, money was tight. After expenses, my first year's income was below the poverty line, and I also had fifteen thousand dollars' worth of school and business debt. We were also reeling under in-law problems.

As I've said, our marriage nearly crumbled under that pressure. Then, of all things, Brenda announced she was pregnant shortly after our first wedding anniversary.

After Jasen was born, the boy wouldn't sleep at night. We tried every trick, including letting him cry for long periods, sometimes for hours. Our discouragement was nearly debilitating. Confused, Brenda couldn't take another blow. Life hadn't turned out as we'd hoped, and I didn't have a cherishing heart nearly often enough.

Gratefully, I'd recently made my "eat gravel" stand with God in front of the refrigerator. Reading about Uriah for the first time, I began to see Brenda in a new way. I began to cherish her, despite our difficult circumstances and despite her emotional inability to carry her weight. I began to treat her with tenderness, holding her dear in spite of my feelings. I decided to get up with my son every time he awoke at night, even though Brenda didn't work outside the home after Jasen was born. Logically, since she didn't work and could rest at different times during the day, she should have been the one to get up. By some standards, I should have said, "C'mon, you're a big girl now. Pull yourself up by your bootstraps and get tough!" But she was married to me, and she was my little ewe lamb. I cherished her, helping her out when she needed it most. Perhaps you're wondering how I could do all that under those circumstances? I could do it all because I didn't focus on those *conditions;* I chose instead to focus on the *promises* I'd made as her husband and as a child of God. I cherished her because I'm called to sacrifice my feelings for the sake of hers. I cherished her because I'm to be concerned for her needs first. In short, I cherished her because it was right. And since right feelings normally follow right actions, a restoration of my own tender feelings for her soon followed.

A Promise

During that same period, I noticed a peculiar thing. The physical drain of nursing, the unsettled sleep at night (she would get up and nurse, then hand Jasen to me), and the psychological exhaustion wasted Brenda. If she awoke in the morning and stumbled down to a dirty kitchen, she was immediately discouraged and had difficulty starting her day. As her courage melted, she found it easier to just stay in her pajamas all day. Life seemed dark and dreary.

I didn't like my ewe lamb to start her day this way. Yes, I could have asked Brenda to shape up, grit her teeth, and push harder. I could have reminded her that she wasn't living up to my expectations. Instead, I sacrificed. I made a promise to my wife that I would never go to bed with the kitchen dirty.

I knew what that promise would cost me. Because of her exhaustion, it meant she would often head off to bed and leave me alone to do all the dishes, scrub all the pans, and tidy up the kitchen. It meant that often she would be asleep when I got to bed, and I would miss out on sex. It meant that I would miss out on precious sleep, but I also knew that by doing this, I could cherish my ewe lamb in ways she never thought possible. I never broke my promise.

I cherished Brenda when the feelings weren't there and when my tender, loving feelings returned. Eventually, she grew to be the woman she is today. She's everything I knew she would be. But guess what? She's also more. She saw my cherishing heart and stopped talking divorce. These days, when I speak about God's Word and about loving the unlovely and about living by His standards, I have credibility with her because I've proven myself with her in the most unlovely of times.

Your Song

If cherishing is anything, it's loving your wife for who she is *this* day, not some other day down the line. It's making allowances for all the surprises and inconsistencies that were hidden until life spun her in its new direction.

Your wife has a heart that still beats like a little lamb's heart, a heart that still skips through meadows of hope and desire, longing for love. It may be difficult to see. Maybe her father was an alcoholic or an abuser who didn't protect her. Maybe she isn't much of a Christian. Maybe she was promiscuous before meeting you.

That all may be true. But we know of some other things that are *also* true. In trust to you, she forsook her individual freedom, believing you would provide love and protection. She's still God's little ewe lamb, regardless of the pain and sin she's been through, and He has entrusted her to you.

Every Man's Marriage

We urge you, as you begin building the defense perimeters into your life, to take one more step: pick up and read a copy of *Every Man's Marriage,* a descriptive guide that teaches you how to cherish your wife in a lot more detail than we can offer here. From the beginning, we've intended *Every Man's Marriage* to be read together with *Every Man's Battle,* as a sort of one-two punch. The two resources work effectively together to help build the kind of strong marriages that can more easily defend us from sexual sin.

Read it once on your own, and then read it again with your wife. She may point out some things you've missed, and that's exactly what you want. She wants the best for you—and the marriage.

Let's move on to part 7, where you'll learn what may happen when purity finally sets into your marriage and how to handle these new developments lovingly as a couple.

Part VII

Restoring Your Sexuality Together

19

Sexuality Breaking Bad

A fter receiving countless emails from readers and after living out this message for another two decades, as well as watching the advances in brain research over these same years, we've realized that a key section was always missing from the first edition of *Every Man's Battle:* how a husband can rebuild his sexual relationship with his wife in the wake of a porn addiction.

Navigating marital intimacy within the covenant of marriage can be complicated and fraught with challenges in the best of circumstances, but once your secret porn addiction is revealed to your wife, the path to a restored sexual relationship can seem hopeless. That's because once you pull away from porn, you may discover that your sexuality is "broken" when it comes to performing sexually with a real, flesh-and-blood woman like your wife.

From Fred: The Root Issue

Today, porn has an intense, debilitating impact upon male sexuality. That wasn't prevalent twenty years ago. Back then, quitting porn and avoiding eye candy *enhanced* your sexual intimacy with your wife. That's what I found out when I went cold turkey from looking at the lingerie ads in newspapers and all the rest of it—the positive effects were practically immediate. While my heightened craving for Brenda capsized our sexual equilibrium for a while, nothing really changed in the bedroom except for the elevated frequency. I had no trace of performance problems, and according to my emails, it's still playing out that way for many men today.

But for many others, exactly the opposite is happening because the pornographic landscape has changed dramatically since then. Canadian psychiatrist Dr. Norman Doidge pointed out in his best-selling classic *The Brain That Changes Itself:*

> Thirty years ago "hardcore" pornography usually meant the *explicit* depiction of sexual intercourse between two aroused partners, displaying their genitals. . . .
>
> Now hardcore has evolved and is increasingly dominated by sadomasochistic themes of forced sex, ejaculations on women's faces, and angry anal sex, all involving scripts fusing sex with hatred and humiliation. Hardcore pornography now explores the world of perversion.[*]

In short, today's raunchier, misogynistic porn, now delivered by an unprecedented access to streaming video, can so degrade a guy's neural sexual pathways that we have an epidemic of erectile dysfunction among men of all ages, even for those in their twenties and thirties. It's become so common that the affliction has an official name: porn-induced erectile dysfunction (PIED).

How can guys in their twenties experience erectile dysfunction? They're at the height of their testosterone levels!

The idea does boggle the mind, but only until you dig into the latest research and discover that this progressive "new porn" essentially misdirects your neural pathways to the wrong pleasure center in your brain. Who is responsible for this?

Well, the late pajama-clad huckster Hugh Hefner started it all. When in 1953 Hef's first *Playboy* magazine hit newsstands, featuring Marilyn Monroe on the cover and a naked Marilyn inside, his "sophisticated" (and now quaint) take on pornography initially shocked everyone. But by the end of the 1960s, there was a tacit acceptance by the culture, and by men in particular, that this type of so-called "soft" porn was okay.

---

[*] Norman Doidge, MD, *The Brain That Changes Itself: Stories of Personal Triumph from the Frontiers of Brain Science* (New York: Penguin, 2007), 102.

From Steve: The Playboy Deception

By the way, I can tell you exactly what that centerfold looks like because it was implanted into my four-year-old brain when I saw it hanging in my grandfather's office. I'll never understand why my very strict Southern Baptist parents thought it was okay for a young boy to see pictures like that, but they were obviously unaware of the damage these pictures deliver.

Gratefully, you have an advantage. If you've read this far, you understand the damages, and while it's far more difficult to protect a young mind today than it was back then, there is simply no excuse for not doing all that you can to defend the children God has put in your care.

But most in our culture remain at a disadvantage because they've been hoodwinked by Hefner and others of his ilk who mainstreamed pornography and decoupled sex from a committed, marital relationship. They passed it off as sexual liberation and declared mission accomplished in their march on our sexuality and our society, which they proclaimed now free from the constraints of our Victorian past.

That sounds high minded and even deserving of our thanks. But all Hefner really did was glorify the objectification and depersonalization of women. The #MeToo movement did not start with movie mogul and womanizer Harvey Weinstein but with a man who wore a burgundy velvet smoking jacket and robe all day long and led us all to believe that he experienced the height of male sexual competency and freedom.

But Hef was a fraud, and those who got close to him knew it. His old girlfriends have spoken out and written of their experiences in bed with the *Playboy* founder, and it's clear that pornography neutered him just like it does every other male. Erectile dysfunction stalked him, and his performance was calculated in seconds, not minutes. On top of that, I once heard a commentator describe his one-on-one meetings with Hef, saying that while hundreds of people were hanging around the pool outside the Playboy mansion, and celebrities were constantly running in and out of the place, what struck him most was the vast, empty loneliness resting in the eyes of this man who supposedly lived every carnal man's dream.

Pornographers deserve no thanks! In fact, we hold the scurrilous "accomplishments" of these so-called liberators in utter contempt. Their mainstreamed porn delivers nothing but addictive chains, an escalation of compulsive sexual behavior, and an eventual *decrease* in our sexual pleasure, especially with our wives.

Culturally, though, they won: we've all been profoundly duped by this mindless, endless tragedy of lies. As a result, we're receiving the most painful emails from wives that we've ever seen, like this one from Malia:

> Early in our marriage, I was not fulfilling my husband sexually, but I educated myself about his body and my own and drastically changed my approach in the bedroom. Sexually, I pursued him actively, but he'd become impotent and could not perform with me. Hundreds of times, I asked him, "Honey, can you please tell me how I can meet your sexual needs?"
>
> He always replied that he was satisfied, but I knew he wasn't. How could he be? I was willing to have sex whenever he wanted and in all kinds of different locations, but he couldn't respond to me.
>
> I wasn't aware of his addiction to pornography at the time, so I was completely confused. Over and over again, I'd ask him, "What is going on in your life? Why aren't you interested in me? Are you using porn? Are you having an affair?" I hated asking those questions, but I had to make sense of all this. It was driving me crazy.
>
> He'd always deny the porn and the affairs, and he merely blamed his sexual problems on the fact that he was getting older. But I didn't buy it. He just wasn't that old.
>
> I eventually discovered the porn, and now I'm convinced that he has been so brainwashed by it that he cannot see my beauty. When we are out together, he sure loves looking at other women any chance he gets, so I know his eyes still work. They just don't work with me.
>
> He doesn't get aroused at all when I wear lingerie or skimpy outfits, and he's not even interested in my naked body. In case you're wondering, I am very beautiful and thin and I take care of myself. There are no beauty problems here.

My question to you is as straightforward as I can make it: when a wife works very hard to meet her husband's sexual needs and he pulls away and is not even aroused by her, what is she to do? I'd give anything to have sex with my husband. He still has sex all the time, but he just won't do it with me. He only wants sex with his porn.

We know exactly what Malia has to do, and we'll share our answer in coming pages. For now, we'll simply take issue with the last line of her email. You see, we disagree that her husband only wants sex with his porn. This implies that he still has a choice in the matter, but it's probably not a choice for him anymore. Most likely, it's become an ability issue, and porn is the only kind of sex that he is capable of having. His sexuality has been broken and desperately needs fixing.

From Fred: Porn Is Never Harmless

Guys have long claimed that porn is a totally harmless form of entertainment, and I did too, except for that one year in middle school when our scout leaders and coaches cautioned us not to masturbate to porn, warning us of a potentially dire impact: "It'll grow hair on your palms."

Looking at pictures of naked women didn't seem so harmless that year. We weren't quite sure whether or not they were kidding, but we were all sure that a hairy palm would be social suicide with the girls, so we kept that little chestnut in mind when it came to peeking at *Playboy*. Over time, we found little evidence of any long-term impact from porn and masturbation, so we dismissed our fears.

Of course, no one had yet heard of neuroplasticity, so it was easy to smirk and think, *Why worry about what I look at with porn? The blood of Jesus covers it all anyway. I won't go to hell! I'm forgiven.* But who knew that the rush of dopamine was a powerhouse neural change agent? Christ's blood can cover your sin, but it doesn't touch the neuroplastic consequences of your sin. *But porn is just pixels on a screen. Nothing I do in the privacy of my home hurts anyone!* We used to say that too. But it *does* hurt someone. Porn hurts you, and from what we're seeing from this erectile-dysfunction epidemic, it's hurting a lot of wives too. Pornography just isn't as harmless as it once seemed.

The Two Pleasure Systems

By now you're probably wondering, *What is it that "breaks" in these cases?* It certainly isn't your penis. Guys with porn-induced erectile dysfunction can still get an erection in front of their computers.

It actually happens within your brain, which we've already described as your largest sex organ. Comprehending how things break down begins with understanding that you have two separate sexual pleasure systems in your brain: the first has to do with exciting pleasure, and the other has to do with satisfying pleasure. The exciting system relates to the appetitive pleasure that you get while imagining something you desire, such as sex with your internet porn. Pornography activates the appetitive system through a large release of dopamine, which raises your sexual tension level and puts your focus on the intensity of the sexual experience.

The second pleasure system has to do with a deep satisfaction, or a consummatory pleasure, that results from having sex with a real-live, flesh-and-blood woman. It's a calming, fulfilling pleasure, and its neurochemistry is based on the release of endorphins, which are related to opiates. This is why you experience a peaceful, euphoric bliss and a deep sense of intimacy with your wife when you make love to her.

Dr. Doidge emphasized these two pleasure centers in *The Brain That Changes Itself* when he pointed out that neuroplastic changes wrought by porn eventually misdirect the focus of our sexuality and adjust our sexual tastes. Here's what he wrote, with our bracketed inserts and italics for emphasis:

> Pornography, by offering an endless harem of sexual objects, hyperactivates the appetitive system [at the expense of the consummatory system, which is meant to be the primary sexual pleasure center]. Porn viewers develop new maps in their brains, based on the photos and videos they see. Because it is a use-it-or-lose-it brain, when we develop a map area, *we long to keep it activated* [which increases and exacerbates our sexual tension]. Just as our

muscles become impatient for exercise when we've been sitting all day, so too do our senses hunger to be stimulated [and we long for another porn session].

The men at their computers looking at porn were uncannily like the rats in the cages of the NIH [National Institutes of Health], pressing the bar to get a shot of dopamine or its equivalent [in their NIH studies meant to measure the strength of certain drugs]. Though they didn't know it, they had been seduced into pornographic training sessions that met all the conditions required for plastic change of brain maps. Since neurons that fire together wire together, these men got massive amounts of practice wiring these images into the pleasure centers of the brain, with the rapt attention necessary for plastic change. They imagined these images when away from their computers, or while having sex with their girlfriends, reinforcing them.[*]

So then, every time these men felt the sexual excitement from these memories or from the masturbation and orgasm over these mental pictures, the reward neurotransmitter dopamine was released, which consolidated the new neural connections being built in the brain's sexual pleasure centers. This dopamine not only rewarded the current bad behavior but also facilitated and expedited any future bad behavior by reinforcing these new pathways.

Doidge continued,

The content of what they found exciting changed as the Web sites introduced themes and scripts that altered their brains *without their awareness*. [The new themes and scripts actually changed their sexual tastes on a neuronal level as well.] Because plasticity is competitive, the brain maps for new, exciting images increased at the expense of what had previously attracted them [which was now fading and decomposing]—the reason, I believe, they began to find their girlfriends less of a turn-on.[†]

---

[*] Norman Doidge, MD, *The Brain That Changes Itself: Stories of Personal Triumph from the Frontiers of Brain Science* (New York: Penguin, 2007), 108–9, emphasis added.
[†] Doidge, *Brain That Changes Itself*, 109, emphasis added.

And that's also why married addicts can't respond sexually to their wives. Their neural maps have transformed their sexual focus away from *intimacy* and toward *intensity*. Remember, internet porn does more than hike the level of dopamine for the sake of a pleasure high. The lewd images literally change the physical structure of the brain so that it *requires pornography* to even generate the reward response, rather than requiring sex with a real woman.

Let's simplify what's actually going on inside the brain by returning to the trains-and-railroads metaphor we used earlier to explain the concept of neuroplastic change. In your brain system of neural rail lines, you have two sexual hubs: one is called Appetitive Station, and the other is called Consummatory Station.

By nature, we know that Consummatory Station is to be your primary sexual hub. After all, God talks in the Bible about sex only in the context of two. That's significant because only two-person sex releases an orgasm that delivers the neurochemistry of satisfaction and intimacy. Clearly, God intended Consummatory Station to be your primary stop with your wife. He even declared that your sexuality doesn't just belong to you but that it also belongs to her (see 1 Corinthians 7:4), which makes it obvious that you don't even have a right to ride out to Appetitive Station alone without her permission.

But somewhere along the way, you discovered that sexual "intimacy" with yourself is much easier than having sex with a real woman. When there's no requirement of intimacy and no real connection with another soul, you needn't concern yourself with *her* sexual needs or *her* pleasure. In the end, what you've done is replace your primary tracks, directing primary travel through Appetitive Station and laying down an even stronger set of rails stretching straight out to nowhere.

When your sexual engines require steeper and steeper climbs to the summit through raunchier and even more perverse levels of porn, you don't mind—or really notice. You keep right on consolidating your tracks until every bit of your sexual stimulation filters back through to your new sexual hub.

But now when your wife draws you gently into her arms to bless you with a slow and passionate kiss, she finds she has no ticket to ride. Your train doesn't stop at her station anymore. The rails to Consummatory Station lie overgrown, desolate and lonely from lack of use, and intimacy's engines are lying useless on their sides, rusting in the rain, having derailed long ago.

But that needn't be the end of your story. You can rebuild the tracks to Consummatory Station and return your wife's ticket to ride, because unlearning and weakening the synaptic connections between neurons is just as plastic a process as laying down the wrong tracks in the first place. That is really great news!

If you're game, let's start tearing up some tracks in the next chapter.

20

From Here to Intimacy

As we saw in the previous chapter, the neuroplastic impact of porn changes your sexual focus from intimacy to intensity and misdirects your sexual neural pathways to Appetitive Station. Perhaps even worse, that same process shifts your sexual tastes at the synaptic level away from your wife.

God perfectly grasps the addictive nature of that appetitive pleasure system with its all-in focus on intensity, but He wants something deeper and better for you: a soul connection that you may not have yet experienced in your life together, even after years of marriage.

How do you get there? The answer is as simple as the use-it-or-lose-it principle: you must stop using the overstimulated, drug-laced synaptic pathways to the wrong pleasure center, and you must start rebuilding your overgrown and deteriorating rails to reach the right pleasure center.

A brief review of the basics of neuroplastic change may be helpful here. Remember, when you quit an activity (like going cold turkey on internet porn and other outside bowls of sexual gratification) and no longer use these neural connections, the synapses in these pathways weaken and eventually fade, break down, and die. The use-it-or-lose-it principle rules the entire neuroplastic process whether you are in the course of learning or unlearning.

Also remember that, based on your conscious decisions regarding your daily behavior and experiences, you can either bolster your synapses or allow them to languish. In other words, you have indirect control over your neural pathways, which is extraordinarily useful in your unlearning process.

Remember how Ethan's brain unlearned what it knew about his daughter Skylar's naptime? He broke his habit of masturbating at noon every Monday through a set of consistent, conscious decisions that allowed him to unlearn those corrupted neural pathways. He deliberately chose to let those synaptic connections weaken, decompose, and die. Like Ethan, you, too, must abandon your corrupted pathways, and it really doesn't matter how corrupted they are. The same use-it-or-lose-it principle applies to those rails to Appetitive Station.

By applying this key principle, you'll unlearn your old focus on intensity when you cut off the porn entirely, which enables the perverted neural pathways to fade from lack of use. You'll also learn a new focus on intimacy as you begin to have sex with your wife rather than with yourself.

How Long Will Healing Take?

Blocking out visual sensuality and unlearning that path to intensity is really what this book is all about. You've already studied how to get your eyes under control, and those defense perimeters impose deep and widespread synaptic changes in your brain. As you take these steps to bounce and starve your eyes, a subconscious wave of synaptic healing unfolds quite naturally, all without further effort from you.

How long does this healing process take?

Well, that's hard to say because there are so many variables. One woman wrote about her husband, saying, "He would try to start something sexually, and then right in the middle he would stop and say, 'I think we should wait!' It drove me crazy, and I would think, *Does he not like me? Is he just toying with me?* It was very confusing until he finally told me about the pornography. He shut down his computer for me, but it still took around nine months for him to hold an erection and perform sexually with me."

This story makes me (Fred) recall a similar conversation that I had with Ben, a local Des Moines business contact. He'd never heard of *Every Man's Battle* before we met, but once he got to know me, he decided to read it. He soon found freedom from a decades-long porn habit.

We're good friends now, and recently we discussed the withering effects of today's hardcore porn and the epidemic of porn-induced erectile dysfunction. As we talked, he admitted that he, too, had been such a victim.

"What happened after you quit the porn, Ben?" I asked.

"It took a very long nine months to get over the effects of the porn, but since then, my wife and I can have regular sex together."

These two anecdotes don't mean that nine months is any kind of magic number, so please don't get hung up on that. We simply thought these real-life examples might give you a feel for the amount of time involved in a restoration.

Once you take the first step (starving your eyes of internet porn), your old sexual maps will naturally degrade over time at their own pace, as the two stories above suggest. But we'd like to suggest an even speedier way to heal. There's a second step that will simultaneously ramp up the construction of *new* rail lines back to the correct pleasure center, Consummatory Station.

Restoring Marital Intimacy

You'll need your wife's help with this step, but before we let you in on the process, let me (Fred) draw your attention back to something in chapter 2 about my early days of dating Brenda. I mentioned that we decided to stay pure before marriage; however, we did kiss, and it was just wonderful! It was my first experience with the paradox of obedience: the physically gratifying payoff resulting from obedience to God's sexual standards. I found that even though I had given up heavy petting and mutual masturbation, which had been my standard operating procedure with women I'd previously dated, I actually got more intimate satisfaction from slowing down and cutting things back with Brenda. A kiss was no longer a joyless prerequisite on the path to intercourse; a kiss had become thrilling again.

We want you to experience the pleasure of this paradox of obedience too. Here's how it works: you can upshift your intimacy with your wife by slowing everything down sexually with her. That certainly looks like a paradox, doesn't it?

Secular counselors would certainly say so. They've been urging their patients for years to do just the opposite to reverse erectile dysfunction: to speed things up by viewing porn with their wives just before bed. Obviously, that is the last thing they should do, given that porn is often the cause of ED these days, not the cure.

Besides, slowing things down is not the paradox it appears to be, at least not from a neuroplastic perspective. Consider this: through the act of slowing things down, you'll end the sexual activities that lit up your old neural maps, which allows them to fade. You'll also be adding simpler, more intimate sexual activities that fire different neurons—neurons that can be wired together and consolidated into new maps tuned toward intimacy.

We call the process skin to skin, and it goes like this. First, find an old television show that you both like—one that has absolutely no sexual content, preferably something funny and cute from an old black-and-white series like *Leave It to Beaver, I Love Lucy,* or *The Dick Van Dyke Show.* These are perfect for your purposes because they're crammed with hilarious, classic humor, but they won't spark a trace of appetitive sexual tension. (Now, if you roll your eyes when it comes to old TV shows in black and white, just hang in there. You'll thank us later.)

Once you and your wife have selected a half-hour episode, take off every stitch of your clothing, spread a blanket on the floor in front of the screen (obviously, you'll choose a private place where the kids won't barge in), and get a pillow for your heads. Do nothing but lie there stark naked as you take in the show. Don't touch each other and don't cover up any part of your bodies with a blanket. Just lie there next to each other giggling and laughing side by side in the nude. You'll be astounded at how much this relaxes you and creates a sense of intimacy and emotional connection.

When the show is over, allow your wife to lie back on her pillow and do nothing but enjoy the next few moments. Begin to stroke her softly, but not in the usual places around her breasts or genitals. Stroke her stomach lightly. Stroke her hair, her shoulders, her thighs, and her calves. Remember, you are not looking to build sexual tension. You're not looking to move quickly toward intercourse. You're looking only for intimacy. You're looking for her.

Frankly, you're just there to listen to her breathe and to listen closely to how she responds to each touch. You are there to connect with her as a person, your precious ewe lamb, and not as a sex partner. Take your time. Slow things down. Caress her. Listen to her responses. Learn of her and from her.

After some time (perhaps fifteen minutes), begin kissing her lips, but *only* her lips, not her breasts and not her neck. Keep your hands at home for now rather than roaming her body's landscape. Keep a single focus, and that is to rediscover the wonder of a kiss. Nothing is more intimate than kissing, not even intercourse. Spend at least ten or fifteen minutes only kissing, slowly and passionately, like you are young lovers again and the clock has been turned back to a more innocent time. Feel her passion. Feel her love for you. Feel her heartbeat.

Let things go wherever they will from there, but take your time. Find *her,* and have sex with *her,* not with her body. You may find that you've never really had sex with her in years.

Skin to skin takes your focus off the sexual event and away from *your* intensity and *your* orgasm. That has to happen if you're to return to true intimacy. With porn, sex had to be about your responses and your climax. No one else was there.

But skin to skin is about *her* responses and *her* climax, which forces your appetitive system to flag and weaken and allows your consummatory system to come alive with satisfying pleasure. This is a time to connect intimately with her and please her, that precious ewe lamb you cherish. As you do, the entire focus of your sexuality will turn back toward intimacy and toward *her* pleasure, and that will remove the mental pressure and your nagging fear of performance issues.

Take the time to experience the paradox of obedience. Let your wife sense your focus on her. Slow down the sex to speed up the unlearning in your brain. We pray that as you do, every one of your corrupted sexual maps will fade and wither.

From Fred: Restoring Your Tastes for Her

In my last two decades of living in sexual freedom, I've discovered certain biblical insights that I couldn't have penned into the original version of *Every Man's Battle* because I didn't yet have the depth of experience and insight. One of these is buried so deeply in Proverbs 5:18–23 that I gleaned it only by chance after living in purity with Brenda over a long period of time:

> Let your fountain (wife) be blessed [with the rewards of fidelity],
> And rejoice in the wife of your youth.

> Let her be as a loving hind and graceful doe,
> Let her breasts refresh and satisfy you at all times;
> Always be exhilarated and delight in her love.

> Why should you, my son, be exhilarated with an immoral woman
> And embrace the bosom of an outsider (pagan)?

> For the ways of man are directly before the eyes of the LORD,
> And He carefully watches all of his paths [all of his comings and goings].

> The iniquities done by a wicked man will trap him,
> And he will be held with the cords of his sin.

> He will die for lack of instruction (discipline),
> And in the greatness of his foolishness he will go astray and be lost. (AMP)

This scripture teaches that your sexual tastes are malleable and they will flex and stretch with your wife's appearance as she ages. That truth isn't easy to spot at first glance, but know this: maintaining visual fidelity to your wife will positively shape your sexual tastes in her favor. God built you this way.

One Pair of Breasts

I didn't see what God was saying here in Proverbs when I was a young husband, probably because my eyes kept locking onto these two lines back then:

Let her breasts refresh and satisfy you at all times;
Always be exhilarated and delight in her love. (verse 19)

Sadly, I always had the same immature response to this passage: *That's easy to do today! But what happens when we're older?* I couldn't imagine later in life being exhilarated sexually by a pair of seventy-year-old breasts, Brenda's or otherwise. I used to just shake my head in dismay, musing, *I guess that is just one more law of God that I'll have to obey by gritting my teeth. Sometimes obedience is easy. Sometimes it's hard.*

Gratefully, over time other parts of this Scripture passage eventually took center stage for me, especially this one:

Why should you, my son, be exhilarated with an immoral woman
And embrace the bosom of an outsider (pagan)? (verse 20)

Once I began building the covenant with my eyes, I noticed that this passage spoke loudly about our visual nature and addictions. If you discipline your eyes to be satisfied only by your *wife's* breasts, you're safe. But if you stray visually and foolishly embrace with your eyes the throngs of young bosoms in cyberspace or elsewhere, you'll be trapped by these immoral women, held fast in addiction by the cords of your sin-built synaptic pathways.

Clearly, disciplining the eyes delivers priceless safety to all of us guys.

But as even more time passed, I discovered that this discipline also releases an even richer blessing from God: you won't have to grit your teeth or force yourself to be exhilarated by your wife as she gets older.

How in the world can this be true?

Easily enough, as it turns out. If you rejoice only in the wife of your youth, and if you let only her breasts satisfy your eyes over the years, your sexual tastes will literally evolve and change along with her aging body. That capacity is already built into you as a man, which means that your obedience today will *enable* you to be exhilarated by your wife in the future, without effort and without a forceful act of your will. It will naturally unfold out of your makeup as a man.

I finally understood that this passage was not so much a command to will ourselves to be thrilled by a pair of seventy-year-old breasts but rather a how-to guide on how to release our innate capacity to do so. Even now, especially if you're under the age of forty, you probably can't quite grasp this, but I think that as you get to see firsthand how God's blessing plays out in an obedient life over time, you'll pick up on it.

A Wicked Roller Coaster

Brenda weighed one hundred thirty pounds when we got married, and that's pretty much where she remained until our fourth and final child was born. That time around, her pregnancy weight did not slip off as easily, and her weight inched up over the years, pound by pound, until at one point she tipped the scales at one hundred ninety-five pounds. (Don't worry—she gave me permission to tell this story.)

Even though Brenda was a full sixty-five pounds heavier than when we married, she was as stunningly sensual to me as she was on our wedding night, and the added weight didn't decrease my sexual passion for her. As for Brenda, she certainly knew that she didn't look the same as she used to, but my natural desire for her did wonders for her self-esteem.

Contrast this to Cody's reaction to his wife's weight gain, as expressed in this email, which echoes a story I've heard from countless other men:

When Michelle and I were married, she was a slender yet full-bodied woman who knocked my socks off! After two years of marriage, however, she started to gain weight. I said some things that hurt her deeply, which just added fuel to the fire. Then she gained even more weight, which sent me into depression.

You see, I'd always pictured my future wife as a slender knockout who I would be not only in *love* with forever but also in *lust* with forever. Once she started packing on more pounds, I began looking at other women in magazines, in movies, and on the internet.

Perhaps you're wondering why Brenda's weight gain didn't affect me the same way. That's easy to answer. Cody's sexual tastes were still tied to young, slender women, and he lusted over magazines, movies, and internet images that fed those tastes. This sexual excitement delivered rewarding releases of dopamine, which consolidated his sexual tastes in the wrong place. Naturally, as Michelle gained weight, his tastes couldn't change along with her.

But I had disciplined my eyes long ago, and I wasn't lusting over young, slender women in the media. My sexual tastes were tied only to Brenda, so as her body changed along life's way, so did my tastes. She was amazed at how passionately I continued to yearn for her.

I've come to love this built-in capacity that alters my sexual tastes as Brenda changes, but that capability has faced the ultimate test in my marriage. Twice, in fact.

When Brenda first tipped the scales at one ninety-five, she decided to go for a checkup. Her doctor discovered that a thyroid problem was the underlying culprit and prescribed medication to balance things out. Brenda began to slowly lose weight.

Right about the time she hit one hundred sixty-five pounds, Brenda received the most traumatic blow of her life: her wonderful mother, Gwen, had been diagnosed with terminal lung cancer and was given less than a year to live.

Brenda's weight plummeted like a boulder rolling off Yosemite's Half Dome, falling forty pounds in about three weeks. The horrific stress of her mother's failing health had jacked her metabolism into the stratosphere, chewing away those extra pounds. By the time she dipped to one hundred twenty-six pounds, Brenda had gone overnight from being a full-bodied, curvy knockout to looking like a wispy, anorexic prepubescent girl.

Let me give you an idea of just how jarring this weight loss was to me as her husband. One morning I woke up groggy after a long night of restless sleep. Swinging my feet out of the bed and onto the floor, I stared straight ahead at our bedroom wall in a dull, vacuous stupor. I heard a soft sound to my left. Glancing over blearily, I glimpsed the profile of a total stranger in her bra and panties standing near the bed, preparing to pull her jeans up her legs.

A silent scream ripped across my soul. *Oh, no! What have I done?*

In my stupor, I was sure my life was ruined. Just as suddenly, though, the shock and awe of the moment torched my senses to full alert and I became fully awake and realized who that stranger really was. *Oh, thank God! It's Brenda!*

That's how drastically Brenda had changed in appearance. Now imagine how strikingly different that body felt to me under the covers at night.

Her abrupt transformation had a startling impact on my sexual senses. As this willing woman pressed her body into mine, she felt nothing like Brenda but more like an utter stranger. I had genuine difficulty responding to her sexually, and at times it felt like a dicey proposition to even get an erection. I never actually failed, but the fears were playing in my mind.

How could that be? She was thin as a supermodel, and isn't that every guy's dream?

This unexpected development hit me with the truth in a fresh way: our sexual tastes are *not* hardwired but are as plastic as the rest of our brains. In fact, I coined a principle at the time that has now been backed up by brain research: *you'll become sexually attracted to whomever you're having sex with on a regular basis.*

Think about it. For years, I'd been making love to a wonderfully curvy, full-bodied woman who drove me crazy with passion. I was not having visual foreplay with every thin, athletic coed in a sports bra who happened across my path. I was not having masturbatory trysts with slender movie starlets after watching their movie bedroom scenes. In short, there was no regular sex for me that would maintain my tastes for shapely, young women.

When a thin babe was thrust into my bed without warning, I couldn't perform up to my normal standards. She wasn't attractive to me—at least not yet. I needed time to adjust, and after a month or two of having sex with a slimmer, leaner Brenda, my tastes morphed again.

A few years later, however, Brenda's thyroid failed further, and the medication became less effective. She took that slow, familiar path up to one hundred ninety pounds. This time I had no problem adjusting my tastes, because the gain was so slow that she remained thrilling to me throughout the climb.

Then disaster struck again. Out of the blue, Brenda was flattened by a severe back issue with searing sciatic pain stabbing down through her left leg and into her toes. Standing up was excruciating. Lying down was excruciating. She could only fitfully sleep by sitting at the kitchen table with her head in her hands. Nights lasted forever, and her days were interminable. Enter Stress Diet 2.0, which torched weight off like butter melting in a skillet. She was one hundred thirty-five pounds in no time flat. We saw specialist after specialist for four dreary months, and no one could find the cause of her pain. We were just a week away from a spinal fusion surgery when the condition vanished overnight. Her pain was gone as quickly as it had come.

Sex resumed, and guess what? The exact same performance fears began wracking my mind. Since Brenda was back down to one hundred thirty-five pounds, I was sleeping with a stranger again. It took a couple of months of having sex with the new Brenda to get completely comfortable in bed again.

After this second time through the wringer, I finally began to understand what God was trying to say to us in Proverbs 5:18–23. Don't forget, I hadn't masturbated in years. I hadn't ogled cute women in my workplace in years. I hadn't even been surfing the web for sensual photo spreads of young actresses.

Every last bowl of sexual gratification was being served up by Brenda. I was allowing only *her* breasts to refresh and satisfy me. I was never visually embracing the bosoms of other women, and because of that, I was able to be exhilarated by Brenda, no matter her weight, no matter her age. When I had eyes only for Brenda, I knew my sexuality would change along with her because God had built within me the capacity for my tastes to follow her lead.

God is so good! The malleability of our sexual tastes is a priceless gift. Perhaps the biggest blessing is that it removes the visual side of our sexuality from the marital equation, allowing us to connect more easily with the soul residing *inside* her body, which is nothing more than a fading tent anyway. According to the apostle Paul, "While we are in this tent, we groan and are burdened, because we do not wish to be unclothed but to be clothed instead with our heavenly dwelling, so that what is mortal may be swallowed up by life" (2 Corinthians 5:4).

You see, you're not to be having sex with her "tent" anymore. You're to have sex with what's inside: her soul and spirit. Her tent, like yours, has fading glory.

Have you ever seen those one-man tube tents online? That's essentially what your body is. Though you are visual, as a man you are not to be focused on tents or to be having sex with a tent alone; you're supposed to be having sex with the wonderful human soul *inside* your wife's tent.

I rejected this strange, obsessive tent world long ago when I engaged the battle for purity. As a result, when I look at Brenda today, I don't see her tent anymore; I see her.

Oh, sure, Fred.

Why does this surprise you? Are you obsessed with your wife's tent, obsessed with her weight and cup size? Perhaps you're depressed when the measurements fall outside your taste parameters. If so, you've been bewitched, and the Lord insists that you change your thinking: "I tell you this, and insist on it in the Lord, that you must no longer live as the Gentiles do, in the futility of their thinking" (Ephesians 4:17).

Look, I'm a guy. I'll be visual until the day I die. But for too many of us, our sexuality is dominated by our eyes, even after we learn to bounce our gaze and stop seeking gratification outside marriage. While we would never say it to our wives, our attitude is clear: *Okay, I've gotten my eyes under control, and you are looking better than ever before! I've done my part. I've gotten rid of my porn stash and stopped looking at the hotties in their thong bikinis. But you have to do your part, babe. Become one of them! Always thin. Always available. Always smiling with that come-on look, ready for action. Become what I've given up for you!*

In fact, some Christian authors are essentially instructing wives to become porn stars for their husbands, insisting it's a woman's responsibility to become what her husband has given up seeking elsewhere for his visual pleasure.

Look, I don't have a problem with you and your wife learning new skills in the bedroom. Ed and Gayle Wheat's classic book *Intended for Pleasure* was immeasurably helpful to Brenda and me when we were first married and learning how to please each other physically. If you've never read a book like this together, you should.

But let me ask you a question: Does making your wife a porn star take you in the right direction? If you need to tear up the tracks to Appetitive Station and get back to God's original plan for intimacy at Consummatory Station, how can this plan possibly help you get there? After all, when doing that, you are still running the same old rails to intensity's playground, consolidating your focus there with the help of dopamine's rewards. You've merely changed which porn star you're viewing. Are you truly connecting intimately with your wife, God's precious daughter, heart to heart? Or are you still just pursuing your fantasies, using your wife as a prop?

The problem with this approach is that there's been no underlying transformation of our corrupted sexuality. It's still not focused on our wives. It's still not about making a cherishing inner connection. It is still only about outer beauty and fantasies and getting our pleasure through our eyes. If our wives don't cut it, will we turn away and look elsewhere for the beauty and thrills? That doesn't seem like a godly response.

There is nothing wrong with outer beauty, but it shouldn't dominate our sexuality, and neither should our eyes, especially since the plasticity of our brain allows our tastes to flex and mold to our wife, if we'll only set our heart to let it happen. God has commanded you to always be ravished by the wife of your youth, but that is not possible if you keep lusting over buxom young babes.

If you *stop* lusting, however, God has something better waiting for you: a wonderful partner you can grow old with and who can continue to satisfy you, even into the golden years. If you allow your tastes to change by walking in His truth and staying disciplined with your eyes, you will be ravished by the wife of your youth until the end of your lives.

Brenda is more sensual to me today than ever before because I'm no longer having sex only with her tent. I'm meeting up with that lovely, ravishing woman inside who displays "the unfading beauty of a gentle and quiet spirit" (1 Peter 3:4).

Gratefully, God has also provided *you* with a wonderful design, including your plastic brain and your malleable sexual tastes. Get disciplined with your eyes and allow God's design to play its proper part in your marriage. It'll free you, and you'll be ravished by your wife's soul every day of your life.

So now go out and make it happen.

Workbook

Questions You May Have About This Workbook

What will the *Every Man's Battle Workbook* do for me? This workbook will guide you through some serious Bible study, an intense examination of your personal life, and an honest application of biblical truth to help you win the war on sexual temptation and live a pure life God's way.

You'll find realistic help straight from God's Word for actively training your eyes and your mind to increasingly see and think according to God's standards. We believe that completing the workbook is critical to the application and absorption of the material in the book *Every Man's Battle.*

The lessons look long. Do I need to work through everything in each one? This workbook is designed to promote your thorough exploration of all the content, but you may find it best to focus your time and discussion on some sections and questions more than on others.

To help your pacing, we've designed the workbook so it can most easily be used in either an eight-week or twelve-week approach.

- For the eight-week track, simply follow along with the basic organization already set up with the eight different weekly lessons.
- For the twelve-week track, lessons 2, 4, 5, and 6 can be divided into two parts (you'll see the dividing place marked in the text).

(In addition, of course, you may decide to follow at a different pace—faster or slower—whether you're going through the workbook individually or as part of a group.)

Above all, keep in mind that the purpose of this workbook is to help guide you in specific life application of the biblical truths taught in *Every Man's Battle.* The wide scope of questions included in each weekly study are meant to help you approach this practical application from different angles and with personal reflection and self-examination. Allowing adequate time to prayerfully reflect on each question will be much more valuable for you than rushing through the workbook.

How do I bring together a small group to go through this workbook? You'll get far more out of this workbook if you're able to go through it together with a small group of like-minded men. And what do you do if you don't know of any group that's going through this workbook? Start such a group of your own!

If you take a copy of this book and show it to the Christian men you know, you'll be surprised at how many will indicate interest in joining you for exploring this topic together. And it doesn't require a long commitment from them. The workbook is clearly set up so you can complete one lesson per week and finish in only eight weeks—or, if you'd like to proceed at a little slower pace, you can follow the instructions provided for covering the exact same content in a twelve-week track.

Your once-per-week meeting could happen during the lunch hour one day at work, in the early morning before work begins, on a weekday evening, or even on a Saturday morning. The location could be an office or meeting room at work, a room at a club or restaurant, a classroom at church, or someone's basement or den at home. Choose a location where your discussion won't be overhead by others so the men are comfortable in sharing candidly and freely.

This workbook follows a simple design that's easy to use. First, each man in the group completes a week's lesson on his own. Then when you come together that week, you all discuss the group questions provided under the "Every Man's Talk" heading in each week's lesson. Of course, if you have time, you can also discuss at length any of the other questions or topics in that week's lesson—we guarantee that the men in your group will find these worth exploring. And they're likely to have plenty of their own related questions to bring up for discussion.

It's best if one person in your group is designated as the group's facilitator. This person is *not* a lecturer or teacher but simply has the responsibility to keep the discussion moving and ensure that each man in the group has an opportunity to fully join in.

At the beginning, remind the men of the simple ground rule that anything shared in the group *stays* in the group—everything's confidential. This will help everybody feel safer about sharing honestly and openly in an environment of trust.

Finally, we encourage you during each meeting together to allow time for prayer—conversational, short-sentence prayers expressed in honesty before God. Many men don't feel comfortable praying aloud before others, so in an understanding way, do all you can to help them overcome that barrier.

1

Where We Are

This week's reading assignment:
the introduction and chapters 1–3 in *Every Man's Battle*

Before you experience victory over sexual sin, you're hurting and confused. *Why can't I win this battle?* you snarl in frustration. As the fight wears on and the losses pile higher, you may begin to doubt everything about yourself, perhaps even your salvation. At best, you think that you're deeply flawed; at worst, an evil person. You probably feel very alone, since men rarely speak openly about these things.

But you're not alone. Countless men have fallen into their own sexual pits, as you are about to see.

—from chapter 3 in *Every Man's Battle*

Every Man's Truth
(Your Personal Journey into God's Word)

As you begin this study, ask for the Holy Spirit's help in hearing and obeying His personal words for you. Read and meditate on the following Bible passages, which have to do with God's holiness and His call to purity. Let the Lord remind you that He is calling you to purity because He has your best interests at heart. Also remember that He delights in you as one who is made in His image and growing into His likeness day by day.

> You have heard that it was said, "You shall not commit adultery." But I tell you that anyone who looks at a woman lustfully has already committed adultery with her in his heart. (Matthew 5:27–28)

> Who will bring any charge against those whom God has chosen? It is God who justifies. Who then is the one who condemns? No one. Christ Jesus who died—more than that, who was raised to life—is at the right hand of God and is also interceding for us. Who shall separate us from the love of Christ? Shall trouble or hardship or persecution or famine or nakedness or danger or sword? . . .
>
> No, in all these things we are more than conquerors through him who loved us. For I am convinced that neither death nor life, neither angels nor demons, neither the present nor the future, nor any powers, neither height nor depth, nor anything else in all creation, will be able to separate us from the love of God that is in Christ Jesus our Lord. (Romans 8:33–35, 37–39)

> "Come now, let us settle the matter,"
>   says the LORD.
> "Though your sins are like scarlet,
>   they shall be as white as snow;
> though they are red as crimson,
>   they shall be like wool." (Isaiah 1:18)

1. What do Jesus's words tell you about His deep concern for your thought life?
2. What comfort do you take in Paul's words to the Roman believers? How does this passage relate to your feelings of guilt when you've given in to lust?

3. When it comes to a believer's sin, how would you distinguish between rebellion and immaturity? What is God's attitude toward us as we grow—and as we stumble—in our attempts to walk in holiness with Him? (Think about your relationships with your own children, if you have them.)

4. "White as snow" is the prophet's imagery for God's holiness. To what extent do you long for holiness and purity in your life? How are Isaiah's words hopeful to you?

Every Man's Choice
(Questions for Personal Reflection and Examination)

You're in a tough position. You live in a world awash with sensual images available twenty-four hours a day in a variety of mediums: print, television, video, the internet, and smartphones.

After teaching on the topic of male sexual purity in Sunday school in the late 1980s, I was approached one day by a man who said, "I always thought that since I was a man, I would not be able to control my roving eyes. I didn't know it could be any other way."

5. Why do you think pursuing sexual integrity is such a controversial topic? How realistic is this pursuit for you?

6. How aware are you of the sensual images all around you? What has been your way of dealing with—or *not* dealing with—this bombardment of sexuality on a daily basis?

7. Have you ever considered your roving eyes to be uncontrollable? In the past, when have you been most likely to lose control? What has helped you to exercise control?

Every Man's Walk
(Your Guide to Personal Application)

———

Steve: I can't tell you what her face looked like; nothing above the neckline registered with me that morning. My eyes feasted on this banquet of glistening flesh as she passed on my left, and they continued to follow her lithe figure as she continued jogging southbound. Simply by lustful instinct, as if mesmerized by her gait, I turned my head further and further, craning my neck to capture every possible moment for my mental video camera.

Then *blam!*

I might still be marveling at this remarkable specimen of female athleti- cism if my Mercedes hadn't plowed into a Chevy Chevelle that had come to a complete stop in my lane.

Fred: There was a monster lurking about, and it surfaced each Sunday morn- ing when I settled into my comfy La-Z-Boy and opened the newspaper. I would quickly find the department-store inserts and begin paging through the colored newsprint filled with models posing in bras and panties. Always smiling. Always available. I loved lingering over each ad insert. I rationalized to myself, *It's wrong, but it's such a small thing! Besides, it's a far cry from* Playboy, *right? And haven't I already given that up?*

So every Sabbath, I peered through the panties, fantasizing.

———

8. How common do you think these situations related by Steve and Fred are among the Christian men you know?

9. Think about Steve's car wreck for a moment. How much trouble have your own eyes gotten you into over the years? What especially painful incident stands out to you at the moment?

10. Fred's eyes were particularly vulnerable to the sensual newspaper ads. In what

situations are your own eyes the most vulnerable? What steps have you taken so far to avoid such situations?

11. Recall that in chapter 2, Fred speaks of the price he was paying for his sin in his relationship with God, with his wife, with his children, and with his church. In which of these areas of life do you think a man's sexual sin hurts him most quickly and obviously? How is it with you?

12. In quietness, review what you have written and learned in this week's study. If further thoughts or prayer requests come to your mind and heart, you may want to write them down.

13. a. What for you was the most meaningful concept or truth in this week's study?

    b. How would you talk this over with God? Write your response down as a prayer to Him.

    c. What do you believe God wants you to do in response to this week's study?

Every Man's Talk
(Constructive Topics and Questions for Group Discussion)

Key Highlights from the Book for Reading Aloud and Discussing

---

When we're fractionally addicted, we surely experience powerful and seemingly irresistible addictive drawings, but we aren't generally compelled to act to salve some pain, at least not in the same intensity as the men at those higher levels of addiction. Instead, we're more compelled by the chemical high and the sexual gratification it brings.

That is telling, isn't it? And it can mean only one thing. There must be something *inside* our makeup as men that makes us particularly susceptible to sexual addiction, and there must be something *outside* us in our culture that makes this whole slippery slope so slick.

If we are ever going to get free, we must first explore our makeup as men and why our sensual culture is so compelling to us in spite of our love for Christ. Only then will we be able to defend ourselves from sexual addiction.

_____

Discussion Questions

A. Which parts of chapters 1–3 in *Every Man's Battle* were most helpful or encouraging to you and why?

B. Which elements of Steve's and Fred's stories made the deepest impression on you? Why?

C. How would you summarize the difference between normal sexual desire and addictive sex?

D. Do you agree that sex can be a way of trying to escape inner pain? What is your own experience with this?

E. Why do you think that sexual sin creates a barrier to intimate worship of God?

F. How would you explain to another man what the authors define as fractional addiction?

G. To what extent do you agree or disagree with the book's contention that for most men, sexual sin is based on pleasure highs rather than true addiction?

H. What aspects of our oversexualized culture that you encounter on a daily basis do you find particularly hard to deal with?

2

How We Got Here (Part A)

This week's reading assignment:
chapters 4–5 in *Every Man's Battle*

For most of us men, becoming ensnared by sexual sin happens easily and naturally, like slipping off an icy log. Why is that? . . .

Most guys expect to grow out of sexual temptation as naturally as they grew into it—like outgrowing acne. Perhaps you waited with each birthday for your sexual impurity to clear up, like I did. But that never happened.

Later, perhaps you assumed that marriage would naturally free you, without a battle. But—as for many of us—that didn't happen either.

—from chapter 4 in *Every Man's Battle*

Every Man's Truth
(Your Personal Journey into God's Word)

Read and meditate on the following Bible passages, which deal with God's judgment and mercy—a combination powerfully demonstrated at the Cross of Christ. There, God's *judgment* upon sin *mercifully* freed us from having to experience sin's destruction. As you study, remember that God's plan is to set sinners free and then use them to teach others.

Follow God's example, therefore, as dearly loved children and walk in the way of love, just as Christ loved us and gave himself up for us as a fragrant offering and sacrifice to God.

But among you there must not be even a hint of sexual immorality, or of any kind of impurity. . . .

For you were once darkness, but now you are light in the Lord. Live as children of light (for the fruit of the light consists in all goodness, righteousness and truth) and find out what pleases the Lord. (Ephesians 5:1–3, 8–10)

It is God's will that you should be sanctified: that you should avoid sexual immorality; that each of you should learn to control your own body in a way that is holy and honorable, not in passionate lust like the pagans, who do not know God; and that in this matter no one should wrong or take advantage of a brother or sister. The Lord will punish all those who commit such sins, as we told you and warned you before. For God did not call us to be impure, but to live a holy life. (1 Thessalonians 4:3–7)

Have mercy on me, O God,
    according to your unfailing love;
according to your great compassion
    blot out my transgressions. . . .
Restore to me the joy of your salvation
    and grant me a willing spirit, to sustain me.
Then I will teach transgressors your ways,
    so that sinners will turn back to you.
    (Psalm 51:1, 12–13)

1. What does Christ's self-sacrifice mean to you? How is it a compelling motive for holy living?

2. What does it mean for you, personally, to live as a child of the light? How can you tell when you're becoming vulnerable to the darkness?

3. How do you respond to the prospect of punishment for sin? In the past, what has been the best motivator or encourager to keep you from sexual impurity? What have you been doing to strengthen this motivation in your life?

4. First offer the words of Psalm 51 to God as a heartfelt prayer of your own. Then take a moment to envision how God might use you in the future to minister to another man regarding sexual purity.

Every Man's Choice
(Questions for Personal Reflection and Examination)

_____

When Mark signed up for my premarriage class, he told me, "The whole problem of impurity has been a mess. I've been hooked for years, and I'm counting on marriage to free me. I'll be able to have sex whenever I want it. Then Satan won't be able to tempt me at all!"

When Mark and I got together a few years later, I wasn't surprised to hear that marriage hadn't fixed the problem. "You know, Fred, my wife doesn't desire sex as often as I do," he said. . . . "I don't want to seem like a sex addict or anything, but I probably have as many unmet desires now as I did before marriage."

So, you haven't naturally grown out of your sexual sin, and marriage hasn't solved your problem either. . . .

Look, it's time you dump the false hopes and accept the truth. . . . If you're tired of sexual impurity and the mediocre, distant relationship with God that results from it, quit waiting on marriage or some hormone drop to save the day.

_____

5. If you were Fred in the conversation above, how would you respond to Mark?

6. Do you agree that marriage isn't necessarily the cure for sexual impurity? What are the practical implications of this for you?

7. If you've been involved in sexual impurity, how have you experienced the distant relationship with God referred to by the authors?

8. What kinds of diluting attitudes or actions have you exhibited over the years?

Every Man's Walk
(Your Guide to Personal Application)

_____

If you're tired of sexual impurity and the mediocre, distant relationship with God that results from it, quit waiting on marriage or some hormone drop to save the day.

If you want to change, you'll have to fight for it. Freedom is never free. Purity will cost you something. You'll need to man up, find your vulnerabilities, and then defend against them with all your heart. Expect a battle. That's the road back to the summit.

It is holy and honorable to completely avoid sexual immorality—to repent of it, to flee from it, and to put it to death in our lives as we live by the Spirit. We've spent enough time living in passionate lust like pagans. It's time to change.

_____

9. What kinds of hidden prices have you paid by failing to be pure with your sexual desires? (Take a moment to sit quietly with your regret and sadness over this. Invite the Lord's presence as you experience this pain.)

10. If you are married, what has surprised you about your sexual experiences with your spouse?

11. Prayerfully consider what it will take for you to completely avoid sexual immorality in the weeks and years ahead. (Think about any changes in your self-image and/or God-image that may be required. Also consider what forms of accountability you may need to establish.)

12. In quietness, review what you have written and learned in this week's study. If further thoughts or prayer requests come to your mind and heart, you may want to write them down.

Every Man's Talk
(Constructive Topics and Questions for Group Discussion)

Key Highlights from the Book for Reading Aloud and Discussing

_____

Sex has different meanings to men and women. Men primarily receive intimacy just before and during intercourse. Women gain intimacy through touching, sharing, hugging, and communication. Is it any wonder that the frequency of sex is less important to women than to men?

Larry found Linda to be far more interested in her career than in fulfilling him sexually. Not only was she disinterested in sex, but she often used it as a manipulative weapon to get her way. Consequently, Larry didn't have sex very often. Twice a month was a bonanza, and once every two months was the norm.
    What's Larry supposed to say to God?

We're not helpless victims here. The truth is, as men we've simply *chosen*, consciously or subconsciously, to mix in our own standards of sexual conduct with God's standard. Somewhere along the way, God's standard felt unnatural or too difficult, so we created a softer, gentler mixture—something new, something comfortable, something mediocre.

_____

Discussion Questions

A. Which parts of chapter 4 in *Every Man's Battle* were most helpful or encouraging to you and why?
B. Do you agree with the authors' description of how sex has different meanings to men and women? (Optional: How would you add to or modify their description to make it more relevant to your situation?)
C. Answer the question that comes at the end of Larry's story: What is he

supposed to say to God? If you were Larry's best friend, how would you counsel him?

D. If a man has mixed his sexuality standards with God's, what first steps can he take to get back on track? (Brainstorm together about practical actions a man can take based upon your experience and/or study so far.)

E. In your own words, and in a practical way that would be helpful for Christian men today, how would you summarize God's standards for sexual purity?

Note: If you're following a twelve-week track, save the rest of this lesson for the following week. If you're on the eight-week track, then keep going.

Every Man's Choice
(Questions for Personal Reflection and Examination)

Excellence is a mixed standard, not a fixed standard. . . .

Is it ever truly profitable for Christians to stop short at this middle ground of excellence? You know, that place where social costs are low and you can live balanced somewhere between paganism and obedience? The answer: *Never!* Sure, in business it may be profitable to *seem* perfect, but in the *spiritual* realm, it's only *comfortable* to seem perfect. It is never profitable spiritually. . . .

As Christ followers, we must shoot for the fixed standard of obedience if we're to ever find sexual freedom.

If you don't kill every hint of immorality—even those that are common—you'll be captured by your tendency as a male to draw sexual gratification and chemical highs through your eyes, and your mixed standards will play right into the Enemy's hands.

But you can't deal with your male eyes until you first deal with your S-type brain and reject your right to mix your standards. As you ask, "How holy can I be?" you must pray and commit to a new relationship with God, fully aligned with His call to obedience.

———————

13. How would you explain the difference between (a) the pursuit of excellence and (b) the pursuit of perfection (through obedience)?

14. Do you believe you have a right to at least sometimes mix your own standards with God's?

15. Consider the difference in attitude reflected in the following questions: (a) How far can I go and still be called a Christian? (b) How holy can I be? How would these attitudes likely manifest themselves in a man's actions?

Every Man's Walk
(Your Guide to Personal Application)

———————

He doesn't want His children to have just His DNA; He wants us to have His character too. I would've never developed His character by hanging around that middle ground, pondering, *How far can I go and still look Christian enough?* To reach maturity, I needed to be asking a different question: *How holy can I be?*

In so many areas, we're often sitting together on the middle ground of excellence, a good distance from God. When challenged by His higher standards, our S-type brains take over subconsciously behind the scenes. We're comforted that we don't look too different from those around us. Trouble is, we don't look much different from non-Christians either.

———————

16. How would you respond to someone who asks, "Why should I eliminate every hint of sexual impurity?"

17. Think through some of the impure temptations and/or practices you've been able to eliminate from your days so far. What hints still remain?

18. Realistically, what is it costing you these days to be a Christian? Make a list of some of your spiritual price tags. What insight does this list offer?

19. What will likely be the next challenge for you, just over the horizon, when it comes to controlling your eyes and mind? What preparations have you made in order to be ready for the onslaught of temptation?

20. a. What for you was the most meaningful concept or truth in this week's study?

   b. How would you talk this over with God? Write your response down as a prayer to Him.

   c. What do you believe God wants you to do in response to this week's study?

Every Man's Talk
(Constructive Topics and Questions for Group Discussion)

Key Highlights from the Book for Reading Aloud and Discussing

---

What is your aim in life—excellence or obedience? What's the difference? To aim for obedience is to aim for perfection and not for excellence, which is actually something less. Your answer to this question reveals whether your spirit or your status-focused male brain is doing your thinking for you.

Your answer also discloses which culture owns your heart: Christ's kingdom culture or the worldly one.

Excellence is deceptive. It helps us sound good and comfortably fit in with the crowd rather than pay the price of true obedience.

Sexual impurity has become rampant in the church because, as individuals, we've ignored the costly work of obedience to God's standards.

If you don't kill every hint of immorality—even those that are common—
you'll be captured by your tendency as a male to draw sexual gratification and
chemical highs through your eyes, and your mixed standards will play right into
the Enemy's hands.

_____

Discussion Questions

F. Which parts of chapter 5 in *Every Man's Battle* were most helpful or encouraging to you and why?

G. Why is it so much easier to learn about prayer than to pray? To learn about purity than to practice purity? What are some of the high costs involved?

H. Look together at the story of King Josiah in 2 Chronicles 34. Read aloud verse 8 and verses 14–33. How do you see Josiah's example in this passage as a model of obedience? What else is Josiah's example here a model of?

I. When are your eyes most likely to play freely? Talk together about actions or attitudes that help you control your eyes. (Be willing to share what works for you.)

3

How We Got Here (Part B)

This week's reading assignment:
chapters 6–7 in *Every Man's Battle*

You stand before an important battle. You've decided that the slavery of sexual sin isn't worth your love of sexual sin. You're committed to removing every hint of it. But how? Some of your male qualities loom as your own worst enemy.

If we got into sexual sin naturally—partly just by being male—then how do we get out? We can't eliminate our maleness, and we really don't want to.

—from chapter 7 in *Every Man's Battle*

Every Man's Truth
(Your Personal Journey into God's Word)

As you begin this study, ask for the Holy Spirit's help in hearing and obeying His personal words for you. Read and meditate on the following Bible passages, which have to do with God's call to faithfulness in marriage. As you read, realize that God is not calling you to anything that's foreign to Himself. The Scriptures proclaim, over and over again, the Lord's utter faithfulness to you!

You shall not commit adultery. (Exodus 20:14)

This command is a lamp,
    this teaching is a light,
and correction and instruction
    are the way to life,
keeping you from your neighbor's wife,
    from the smooth talk of a wayward woman.

Do not lust in your heart after her beauty
    or let her captivate you with her eyes.

For a prostitute can be had for a loaf of bread,
    but another man's wife preys upon your very life.
Can a man scoop fire into his lap
    without his clothes being burned?
Can a man walk on hot coals
    without his feet being scorched? . . .

But a man who commits adultery has no sense;
    whoever does so destroys himself.
    (Proverbs 6:23–28, 32)

He will cover you with his feathers,
    and under his wings you will find refuge;
    his faithfulness will be your shield and rampart. (Psalm 91:4)

1. What are some of the horrible consequences of lust and adultery? How does a man destroy himself in the arms of another woman?

2. When you think of God's faithfulness to you, what events or circumstances of the past spring to mind? (Spend some quiet moments in thankfulness and praise.)

3. How does it feel to know that God's love is like the warm and close protection that a hen offers its young? How can God's faithfulness act as a "shield and rampart" in your life?

4. How easy or difficult is it for you, after you have fallen to temptation, to immediately move back under God's "wings"? Why?

Every Man's Choice
(Questions for Personal Reflection and Examination)

The male eye can perform sexual foreplay, all on its own. That's right. Without even touching a woman.

We normally think of sexual foreplay as tactile or physical, like caressing or kissing a breast. But foreplay is any sensual action that naturally prepares the body for intercourse, that ignites passion, rocketing us by stages until we want to go all the way. It needn't be tactile. . . .

No doubt about it: for men, visual sexual gratification is a form of sexual foreplay.

I understood better how manhood looks after reading a newsletter by author and speaker Dr. Gary Rosberg. In it, he told of seeing a pair of hands that reminded him of the hands of his father, who had gone on to heaven. Gary continued to reminisce about what his father's hands meant to him. Then he shifted his thoughts to the hands of Jesus, noting this simple truth: "They were hands that never touched a woman with dishonor."

5. Have you ever before considered the dangers of visual foreplay? What is your reaction to the authors' statements about it?

6. What role is visual sexual gratification playing in your life these days? What is your level of awareness of it?

7. Think about the reputation of Jesus's hands for a moment. What legacy will your hands leave behind?

8. Read Galatians 6:7–8. How have you seen the truth of this principle in your own life?

Every Man's Walk
(Your Guide to Personal Application)

I [Fred] remember the moment—the exact spot on Merle Hay Road in Des Moines—when it all broke loose. I'd just failed God with my eyes for the thirty-millionth time by lusting over a jogger. My heart churned in guilt, pain, and sorrow. I suddenly gripped the wheel, and through clenched teeth I yelled out, "That's it! I'm through with this! I'm making a covenant with my eyes. I don't care what it takes, and I don't care if I die trying. It stops here. It stops here!"

I made that covenant and built it brick by brick. Later, Steve and I will show you the blueprint for building that brick wall, but for now, study the simple nature of my breakthrough:

- I made a clear decision.
- I decided once and for all to make a change.

I can't describe how much I meant it. A flood of frustration from years of failure poured from my heart. I'd just had it! I wasn't fully convinced I could trust myself even then, but I'd finally and truly engaged the battle. Through my covenant with my eyes, all my mental and spiritual resources were now leveled upon a single target: my impurity.

In short, I had also chosen manhood. I'd taken on the big battle to rise above my natural male tendencies, and I'd embarked on a great adventure to put the Enemy under my feet.

Was God proud of Job? You bet! He applauded His servant's faithfulness in words of highest praise. . . .

In Job 31:1, we see Job making this startling revelation: "I made a covenant with my eyes not to look lustfully at a young woman."

A covenant with his eyes! You mean he made a promise with his eyes to not gaze upon a young woman? It's not possible! It can't be true!

Yet Job was successful; otherwise, he wouldn't have made this promise: "If my heart has been enticed by a woman, or if I have lurked at my neighbor's door, then may my wife grind another man's grain, and may other men sleep with her" (verses 9–10).

———————

9. Fred had failed "thirty million" times. How many times has it been for you? Do you believe it will take a crisis-point event like Fred's to bring you to a place of choosing covenant making? Why or why not?

10. Have you ever sensed that the grace of God was the only way out of your cycle of failed willpower? How did you respond?

11. What does it mean for you to rest in God's saving grace? How will you know when you are ready to make that your standard response during the toughest temptations?

12. If you were to make a covenant with your eyes right now, how would you write it?

13. In quietness, review what you have written and learned in this week's study. If further thoughts or prayer requests come to your mind and heart, you may want to write them down.

14. a. What for you was the most meaningful concept or truth in this week's study?

    b. How would you talk this over with God? Write your response down as a prayer to Him.

    c. What do you believe God wants you to do in response to this week's study?

Every Man's Talk
(Constructive Topics and Questions for Group Discussion)

Key Highlights from the Book for Reading Aloud and Discussing

_____

Our eyes give us guys the means to sin broadly and at will. We don't need a date or a mistress. We don't need to wait for a woman to drop by our apartment. We have our eyes to call upon, and we can draw genuine sexual gratification through them at any time. We're turned on by female curves and nudity in any way, shape, or form.

"Modern science allows us to understand that the underlying nature of an addiction to pornography is chemically nearly identical to a heroin addiction: Only the delivery system is different, and the sequence of steps." [For the source information, please see page 59.]

This neurological process is incredible, when you think about it. Based on your conscious decisions regarding your daily behavior and experiences, you can either bolster your synapses or allow them to languish. In other words, you have control over your neural pathways, which is extraordinarily useful in your battle for purity.

_____

Discussion Questions

A. Which parts of chapters 6 and 7 in *Every Man's Battle* were most helpful or encouraging to you and why?

B. Males are rebellious by nature. Obviously, this trait is not a gift from God but a result of our sinful nature as fallen human beings. Think about other maleness traits. To what degree is each one a gift from God, and to what degree is each one a result of our sinful nature?

C. How would you describe the difference between maleness and manhood?

D. How do recent discoveries of brain science give new hope to our struggles with sexual lust?

E. Do you totally buy into the conclusion that a real man is one who is a doer of the Word of God? Why or why not?

F. How important is the fellowship of other Christian men when it comes to your ability to be a doer of the Word? What are the opportunities for forming accountability relationships within your group? Talk about it!

4

Choosing Victory

This week's reading assignment:
chapters 8–10 in *Every Man's Battle*

When you talk to courageous . . . World War II veterans who embody the title of Tom Brokaw's book *The Greatest Generation,* they say they simply had a job to do. When the landing-craft ramps fell open, those men swallowed hard and said, "It's time." Time to fight.

In your struggle with sexual impurity, isn't it time? Sure, fighting back will be hard. It was for us. . . .

Your life and home are under a withering barrage of machine-gun sexuality that rakes the landscape mercilessly. Right now you're in a landing craft, inching closer to shore and a showdown. God has given you the weapons and trained you for battle.

You can't stay in the landing craft forever.

—from chapter 8 in *Every Man's Battle*

Every Man's Truth
(Your Personal Journey into God's Word)

As you begin this study, read and meditate on the following Bible passages, which have to do with your identity and power in Christ. Remember that Christ has already fought the battle against sin on your behalf—and won. Now it is time to live in that victory! Ask the Holy Spirit to lead you into specific, practical applications for your daily life.

> Grace and peace be yours in abundance through the knowledge of God and of Jesus our Lord.
>
> His divine power has given us everything we need for a godly life through our knowledge of him who called us by his own glory and goodness. Through these he has given us his very great and precious promises, so that through them you may participate in the divine nature, having escaped the corruption in the world caused by evil desires. (2 Peter 1:2–4)

> If we died with Christ, we believe that we will also live with him. For we know that since Christ was raised from the dead, he cannot die again; death no longer has mastery over him. The death he died, he died to sin once for all; but the life he lives, he lives to God.
>
> In the same way, count yourselves dead to sin but alive to God in Christ Jesus. Therefore do not let sin reign in your mortal body so that you obey its evil desires. Do not offer any part of yourself to sin as an instrument of wickedness, but rather offer yourselves to God as those who have been brought from death to life; and offer every part of yourself to him as an instrument of righteousness. For sin shall no longer be your master, because you are not under the law, but under grace. . . .
>
> You have been set free from sin and have become slaves to righteousness. (Romans 6:8–14, 18)

We take captive every thought to make it obedient to Christ. (2 Corinthians 10:5)

1. According to Peter, what exactly has God given you? What is the source of your ability to "participate in the divine nature"? When have you most powerfully sensed the glory and goodness of Jesus in your life?
2. If we have everything we need for Godliness, what is holding us back from constant, lifelong sexual purity? (Think about what it means to count yourself dead to sin.)
3. In the heat of sexual temptation, what will it mean for you to *not* "offer any part of yourself to sin," as Paul says? What will offering yourself to God require at that point? (Give some thought to the role your willpower can and can't play at this point in the battle.)
4. When are your thoughts typically most "captive"? When are they most likely to roam free?

Every Man's Choice
(Questions for Personal Reflection and Examination)

I was angry too. I was sick of sinning, sick of Satan, and sick of me. I didn't want to wait anymore. Like the people of Israel, I came to loathe myself (see Ezekiel 6:9). I wanted to win right away and to win decisively, not somewhere down the road where aging might bring victory through the back door. I wanted to win when the battle was hottest.

You should too. If you don't win now, you'll never know whether you're a man of God who's truly after His purposes.

Sexual sin isn't just a game out there, just one more form of scintillating entertainment. It warps the pathways to your brain's pleasure centers. It literally changes your sexual tastes, and it will lock you up spiritually and throw away the key. If you're going to engage the battle, know this: you've got to fight for keeps. There will be no victory in this area of your life until you choose manhood and choose victory with all your might.

_____

5. How angry are you about the battle? On a scale of one to ten, how convinced are you that God's will is for you to win the battle and be sexually pure?

6. On a scale of one to ten, to what extent would you say you truly hate the sin of sexual impurity in any form?

7. On a scale of one to ten, to what extent do you truly expect to win the battle for sexual purity? What are your reasons for picking this score?

8. If you see some aspects of the prodigal son within you, where are you in your journey? Are you still heading for adventure in the big, wide world? Suffering loss and desperation? On your way back home?

Every Man's Walk
(Your Guide to Personal Application)

_____

Listen to the following words spoken in a sermon by the late evangelist Steve Hill, who was addressing his personal escape from addiction to drugs and alcohol, as well as from sexual sin: "There's no temptation that is uncommon to man. God will send you a way of escape, but you've got to be willing to take that way of escape, friend."

God is waiting for you. But He is not waiting by the altar at church, hoping you'll drop by for the umpteenth time to cry for a while. He is already out on the battlefield, glancing at His watch, waiting for you to arrive and rise up and engage in the battle. You have the spiritual power through the Lord to overcome every level of sexual immorality, but if you don't stand up and utilize that power, you'll never break free of the habit.

_____

9. What is your strongest motivation for achieving and maintaining sexual purity?

10. Recall some of the times when you gave in to sexual temptation. Was there always a "way of escape" open to you? In a particular instance, what do you think kept you from taking the escape route?

11. Read Romans 12:1–2. Imagine completely giving up sexual fantasy in your life. How much grief would that bring you? Are you ready to experience that pain as an act of sacrificial worship?

12. Who in your life now serves as a spiritual accountability partner? If there's no one, who might be that man for you?

13. In quietness, review what you have written and learned in this week's study. If further thoughts or prayer requests come to your mind and heart, you may want to write them down.

14. As you think of attaining the sexual purity that is God's will for you, how do you envision your relationship with God in the near future? Your relationship with your wife? Your future legacy for your children? Your ministry in the church, both in the near future and long term?

15. a. What for you was the most meaningful concept or truth in this week's study?

   b. How would you talk this over with God? Write your response down as a prayer to Him.

   c. What do you believe God wants you to do in response to this week's study?

Every Man's Talk
(Constructive Topics and Questions for Group Discussion)

Key Highlights from the Book for Reading Aloud and Discussing

---

Sexual impurity isn't like a tumor growing out of control inside you. You treat it that way when your prayers focus on some dramatic spiritual intervention, like deliverance, as you plead for someone to come remove it. Actually, sexual impurity is a series of bad decisions on your part—sometimes as a result of immature character—and deliverance won't deliver you into instant maturity. Character work needs to be done so that the warped synaptic pathways in your brain can die, as grace "teaches us to say 'No' to ungodliness and worldly passions, and to live self-controlled, upright and godly lives in this present age" (Titus 2:12).

Remember this: holiness is not some nebulous, mystical thing. You needn't wait around for some holy cloud to form around you. From the perspective of daily practice, it's simply a series of right choices. You'll be holy when you choose not to sin.

You already have everything you need inside to win this battle. . . . In the millisecond it takes to make that choice, the Holy Spirit will start guiding you and walking through the struggle with you.

After all, it's God's will for you to have sexual purity, though you may not think so since this hasn't been your constant experience.

The power of friendship and intimacy extends even beyond the sharing of tips and insights, as awesome as that is. If you think you don't need connection because you're a real man, we suggest that it is precisely *because* you are a real man that you need connection. As a red-blooded male, you have a weak spot in your sexuality that will always be open to attack when you're disconnected from others, no matter how strong your internal defenses feel today.

You see, it's not just the natural accountability in these relationships that gives connection its strength; it's the intimacy itself.

_____

Discussion Questions

A. Which parts of chapters 8–10 in *Every Man's Battle* were most helpful or encouraging to you and why?

B. What is wrong with praying for deliverance year after year?

C. Describe, as clearly and concisely as you can, the provision God has made for us.

D. Talk in practical terms about what *choosing* means to you.

E. Why does a "real man" need to have a strong connection to another godly man? What keeps men from having such friendships?

F. Take a few moments as a group to reflect silently on these questions as they apply and relate to you: (1) How long are you going to stay sexually impure? (2) How long will you rob your wife sexually? (3) How long will you stunt the growth of oneness with your wife, a oneness you promised her years ago?

> Note: If you're following a twelve-week track, save the rest of this lesson for the following week. If you're on the eight-week track, then keep going.

Every Man's Choice
(Questions for Personal Reflection and Examination)

Satan's greatest weapon against you is . . . deception. He knows Jesus has already purchased your freedom. He also knows that once you see the simplicity of this battle, you'll win in short order, so he deceives and confuses. He whispers, tricking you into thinking you're a helpless victim, someone who'll need years of group therapy.

Your goal is sexual purity. Here's a good working definition of it, good because of its simplicity: *you are sexually pure when you're getting no sexual gratification from anyone or anything but your wife.*

In other words, victory means stopping the sexual gratification that comes into you from outside marriage. . . .

Your objective in the war against lust is to build a three-layered defense perimeter into your life:

1. With your eyes
2. In your mind
3. In your heart

_____

16. Have you ever viewed yourself as a helpless victim to sexual temptation? According to Steve and Fred, what is a more honest assessment?

17. What is your reaction to the authors' definition of *sexual purity*? To what extent are you ready to use this definition in daily practice as you battle for sexual purity?

Every Man's Walk
(Your Guide to Personal Application)

_____

The simple truth? Impurity is a habit. It lives like a habit. When some hot-looking babe walks in, your eyes have the bad habit of bouncing toward her and then sliding up and down. . . .

The fact that impurity is merely a habit comes as a surprise to many men. . . .

If impurity were genetic or some victimizing spell, you'd be helpless. But since impurity is a habit, it can be changed. You have hope because if it lives like a habit, it can die like a habit. For Fred, it took about six weeks to change his eye habits, but admittedly, that is on the short end of normal.

Don't misunderstand—we're not saying your habits have no relationship to your emotions or circumstances. Glen told us, "My sexual sin became much worse when I was under a deadline at work and especially whenever my wife and I fought or I felt unloved and unappreciated. It seemed at those times that I was compelled to sin sexually and couldn't say no."

_____

18. Consider why the authors believe impurity and masturbation are habits. To what extent do you agree or disagree with their reasoning?

19. Think of some habits that you've "killed" in the past. Do you believe the impurity habit can die as well? What gives you hope?

20. a. What for you was the most meaningful concept or truth in this week's study?

b. How would you talk this over with God? Write your response down as a prayer to Him.

c. What do you believe God wants you to do in response to this week's study?

Every Man's Talk
(Constructive Topics and Questions for Group Discussion)

Key Highlights from the Book for Reading Aloud and Discussing

---

Masturbation is the path of least resistance—a pretend lover, a pornographic lover with a permanent smile. A lover who never says no, one who never rejects. One who never abandons and is always discreet. One who supports the man's ego in the midst of his self-doubt, who forever says, "Everything will be okay," no matter how high the pressure goes. This path is a chosen path, a path made available by the impure eyes stoking the sexual fever, providing an unending pool of lovers from which to draw.

Whether or not your battle involves spiritual *oppression,* you will always face spiritual *opposition.* The Enemy is constantly near your ear. He doesn't want you to win this fight, and he knows the lies that so often break men's confidence and their will to win. Expect to hear lies and plenty of them.

The first issue is accountability. For many men who are willing to fight for sexual purity, an important step is finding accountability support in a men's Bible-study group, in a smaller group of one or two other men serving as accountability partners, or by going to counseling.

For an accountability partner, enlist a male friend, perhaps someone older and well respected in the church, to encourage you in the heat of battle. The men's ministry at your church can also help you find someone who can pray for you and ask you the tough questions.

_____

Discussion Questions

G. What are the three defense perimeters the authors say we must build to attain the goal of sexual purity?

H. The authors say, "Satan's greatest weapon against you is . . . deception." What do you think are Satan's more effective lies?

I. What is your experience with seeking love in the wrong places? Do you agree this has been a choice? How does rejection or lost love tend to fuel this choice?

J. Talk together about the trust levels in your group in light of the third quotation above. Discuss some ways you can maintain trust with one another in the area of sexual purity.

K. How many men in your group have an accountability partner? How might an accountability partner be found for any man who does not have one?

5

Victory with Your Eyes

This week's reading assignment:
chapters 11–13 in *Every Man's Battle*

When your eyes become aware of a woman, you must train them to bounce away immediately. (Later, we'll explain how to handle bouncing your eyes with women you know.) Why must the bounce be immediate? After all, a glance isn't the same as lusting, right? If we define lusting as staring openmouthed until drool pools at our feet, then a glance isn't the same as lusting. But if we define lusting as any look that creates that little chemical high, that little pop, then we have something a bit more difficult to measure. . . .

Can you tell us exactly *when* that first look sends the impulse through your synaptic pathways and into the pleasure centers of the brain? . . . This chemical high likely happens earlier in the process and much more quickly than you realize.

—from chapter 11 in *Every Man's Battle*

Every Man's Truth
(Your Personal Journey into God's Word)

Read and meditate on the following Bible passages, which have to do with the marvelous visual aspects of God's creation. Let the Lord bless you as you remember He gave you sight that you might enjoy all the beauty and wonder of this world. The ultimate goal, of course, is that your heart may be lifted up in praise of His awesome power and glory. Why let your eyes pursue less-worthy goals?

> LORD, our Lord,
>   how majestic is your name in all the
>   earth!
>
> You have set your glory
>   in the heavens. . . .
> When I consider your heavens,
>   the work of your fingers,
> the moon and the stars,
>   which you have set in place,
> what is mankind that you are mindful
>   of them,
>   human beings that you care for them?
>   (Psalm 8:1, 3–4)
>
> The heavens declare the glory of God;
>   the skies proclaim the work of his
>   hands.
> Day after day they pour forth speech;
>   night after night they reveal knowledge.
> They have no speech, they use no words;
>   no sound is heard from them.
>   (Psalm 19:1–3)

My eyes are ever on the LORD,

for only he will release my feet from the snare.

(Psalm 25:15)

1. Consider the majesty of God conveyed by the heavens. When have you experienced this awesomeness in a night sky? Give thanks!
2. How can creation "reveal knowledge"? What have you seen of God in nature?
3. If you've been using your eyes more for lust than for worship, what would you like to say to the Lord about that right now? What practical actions might help you keep your eyes "ever on the Lord" this day?

Every Man's Choice
(Questions for Personal Reflection and Examination)

A red-blooded American male can't watch a major sporting event without being assaulted by commercials showing a bunch of half-naked women cavorting on a beach with some beer-soaked yahoos. What's a man to do?

To attain sexual purity as we defined it, you must starve your eyes and phase out the bowls of sexual gratification coming from outside your marriage. When you starve your eyes and eliminate "junk sex" from your life, you'll deeply crave "real food": your wife. And no wonder. She's the only thing in the kitchen cabinet, and you're hungry!

---

4. Think about the red-blooded American male's dilemma in front of the television. What is Fred's solution? Define *bouncing the eyes*.
5. How many bowls of gratification do you think you receive from "junk sex" in a typical day? What will starving the eyes look like for you? And are you ready to crave your wife more deeply?

Every Man's Walk
(Your Guide to Personal Application)

While I [Fred] can't determine the best defense for *your* weaknesses (since I don't know what they are), let me share how I defended my own so you'll get a feel for the process. . . .

Rule 1: When my hand reached for a magazine or insert and I sensed in even the slightest way that my underlying motive was to see something sensual (rather than looking for a sale on tires or landscape timbers, for instance), I forfeited my right to pick up and peruse that week's ad insert, no matter what savings I might have discovered for our household budget.

My body began to fight back in interesting ways. . . .

Whenever another brain trick worked, I'd bark to myself in sharp rebuke, *You've made a covenant with your eyes! You have no right to do that anymore.* In the first two weeks, I must have snarled that at myself hundreds of times, but the repeated confession of truth eventually worked to transform my mind.

---

6. Look over Fred's greatest areas of weakness in chapter 11. What would be on your own list of sources (other than your wife) where you draw sexual satisfaction visually? (Spend plenty of time coming up with an accurate list that doesn't overlook any important areas.)

7. Now take time to come up with defense tactics in each identified area.

8. Fred says he can't define the actual defense methods that will work best for you, but what did you think of his own rules? What about rule number one? What rules are you considering for yourself?

9. Are you ready for your body and mind to fight back, as Fred's did? What forms of inner rebellion will you likely need to prepare yourself for in this battle?

10. In quietness, review what you have written and learned in this week's study. If further thoughts or prayer requests come to your mind and heart, you may want to write them down.

Every Man's Talk
(Constructive Topics and Questions for Group Discussion)

Key Highlights from the Book for Reading Aloud
and Discussing

Imagine that your current level of sexual hunger takes in about ten bowls of sexual gratification per week. These bowls of pleasure should be filled from your single legitimate vessel of sexual fulfillment, the wife God provided for you. But because we can soak up sexual gratification through our eyes, we can effortlessly fill our bowls from other sources.

Wait a minute, Fred, you say. *Cutting down from ten bowls to six bowls seems unfair. If I follow your path, I'll be cheated sexually, all because I'm obeying God!*

I guarantee you won't feel cheated. First, without the constant hyperstimulation of your sex drive from visual binging, your sexual hunger will return to normal, original specs. Second, with your whole sexual being now focused on your wife, sex with her will be so transformed that your satisfaction will explode off any known scale, even while consuming fewer bowls. It's a personal guarantee, backed by the full faith, credit, and authority of the Word of God.

Discussion Questions

A. Which parts of chapters 11 and 12 in *Every Man's Battle* were most helpful or encouraging to you and why?

B. What is your reaction to the bowls analogy? How helpful is it for you to view your sexual need this way? Why?

C. How do you think most wives would respond to a husband who's newly enamored with her? How would you counsel a friend in this situation as he helps his wife learn what's going on?

D. In your opinion, what percentage of men will likely react to starving the eyes with "I'm being cheated"? Why? What is the author's response?

> Note: If you're following a twelve-week track, save the rest of this lesson for the following week. If you're on the eight-week track, then keep going.

Every Man's Choice
(Questions for Personal Reflection and Examination)

You'll need a good Bible verse to use as a sword and rallying point. . . .
   Your shield—a protective verse that you can reflect on and draw strength from even when you aren't in the direct heat of battle—may be even more important than your sword because it helps eliminate temptation and moves it out of earshot.

---

11. Why do you need a sword and shield, according to this chapter? What is their value in your pursuit of sexual purity?

12. What are the merits of the opening line of Job 31 as a sword verse? To challenge this verse, what arguments do you think Satan and his forces would be likely to use?

13. What are the merits of 1 Corinthians 6:18–20 as a shield passage? To challenge this passage, what arguments do you think Satan and his forces would be likely to use?

14. What aspects of the authors' strategy for bouncing and starving the eyes

make the most sense to you? What questions do you still have about these plans?

Every Man's Walk
(Your Guide to Personal Application)

_____

We may fear that temptation will be too strong for us in this battle, but temptation honestly has no power at all without our own arrogant questions and the supposed right to choose our behavior. Once we become Christians, we are no longer to have such choice.

In the long term, . . . do you still have to monitor your eyes? Yes, because the natural bent of your eyes is to sin, and you'll return to bad habits if you're careless. But with only the slightest effort, good habits are permanent. . . .

After a year or so—though it may take longer—nearly all major skirmishes will stop. Bouncing your eyes will become deeply entrenched. Your brain, now policing itself tightly, will rarely slip anymore, having given up long ago on its chances to return to the old days of pornographic pleasure highs.

_____

15. What verses will you select for your sword and for your shield?
16. What are some of the important questions in the realm of sexual temptation that you no longer have a right to ask yourself?
17. What kind of short-term results and reactions do you expect in your pursuit of sexual purity? What kind of long-term results and reactions do you expect in your pursuit of sexual purity?
18. In your own life, what do you believe are the most important factors that will ensure the success of this entire strategy for purity through your eyes?
19. a. What for you was the most meaningful concept or truth in this week's study?
    b. How would you talk this over with God? Write your response down as a prayer to Him.

c. What do you believe God wants you to do in response to this week's study?

Every Man's Talk
(Constructive Topics and Questions for Group Discussion)

Key Highlights from the Book for Reading Aloud and Discussing

---

Once on an overnight hotel stay, I walked down the hallway to the ice machine. On top of the machine was a *Playboy* magazine. Mistakenly believing that I had a right to choose my behavior, I asked myself this question: *Should I look at this* Playboy *or not?*

The moment I asked that question, I opened myself to outside counsel. Sure, I began talking the pros and cons to myself internally, just as my question would suggest. But without noticing it, that question *also* opened myself up to Satan's counsel. He wanted to be heard on this issue. . . .

Therein lies the power of temptation. We may fear that temptation will be too strong for us in this battle, but temptation honestly has no power at all without our own arrogant questions.

Looking back at the details of our plan for your eyes, even we will admit that it all sounds slightly crazy. Defenses, brain tricks, bouncing your eyes, forfeiting rights. Man! We wonder if even Job would be a bit startled.

On the other hand, maybe we should expect a sound plan to look this way. Consider all the men who are called to purity, yet so few seem to know how to make it happen.

Discussion Questions

E. Which parts of chapter 13 in *Every Man's Battle* were most helpful or encouraging to you and why?

F. Have you ever "been there" at the ice machine with Fred? What did you do in a similar situation?

G. According to Fred, what is the problem with getting into a conversation with ourselves about how we should respond to a particular temptation?

H. Fred and Steve admit that their plan for purity may seem slightly crazy. Have you had that reaction during this course of study? Talk about it!

Victory with Your Mind

The great news is that the defense perimeter of the eyes works with you to build the perimeter of the mind. The mind needs an object for its lust, so when the eyes view sexual images, the mind has plenty to dance with. Without those images, the mind has an empty dance card. By starving your eyes, you starve your mind as well.

—from chapter 14 in *Every Man's Battle*

Every Man's Truth
(Your Personal Journey into God's Word)

As you begin this week's study, read and meditate on the following Bible passages, which deal with appreciating God's grace, love, and power. Remember that you can choose to fill your mind with thoughts of God's goodness throughout your day. Think on these things!

Answer me, LORD, out of the goodness
   of your love;
   in your great mercy turn to me.
Do not hide your face from your servant;
   answer me quickly, for I am in trouble.
Come near and rescue me;
   deliver me because of my foes.
   (Psalm 69:16–18)

Praise be to the God and Father of our Lord Jesus Christ, who has blessed us in the heavenly realms with every spiritual blessing in Christ. For he chose us in him before the creation of the world to be holy and blameless in his sight. In love he predestined us for adoption to sonship through Jesus Christ, in accordance with his pleasure and will—to the praise of his glorious grace, which he has freely given us in the One he loves. In him we have redemption through his blood, the forgiveness of sins, in accordance with the riches of God's grace that he lavished on us. (Ephesians 1:3–8)

Brothers and sisters, whatever is true, whatever is noble, whatever is right, whatever is pure, whatever is lovely, whatever is admirable—if anything is excellent or praiseworthy—think about such things. (Philippians 4:8)

1. Have you ever prayed the words of Psalm 69 that King David prayed? Do you have this fellow sinner's confidence in God's goodness, love, and mercy?
2. Meditate on the blessings proclaimed in Ephesians 1:3–8. Make a list of the spiritual riches bestowed upon you as an adopted son of the heavenly Father. How will you live as His son today?
3. To what extent will your mind need transforming if you are to carry out the apostle's command in Philippians 4:8?

Every Man's Choice
(Questions for Personal Reflection and Examination)

Your mind is orderly. The mind will allow these impure thoughts only if they fit the way you look at the world. As you set up the perimeter of defense, your brain's worldview will be transformed by a new matrix of allowed thoughts, or what we call allowables. . . .

This transformation of the mind takes some time as you wait for the old sexual pollution to be washed away. It's much like living near a creek that becomes polluted when a sewer main breaks upstream. After repair crews replace the cracked sewage pipe, it still takes some time for the water down-stream to clear.

Have you "lurked at your neighbor's door"? It could mean stopping by in the late afternoon and visiting your friend's wife for coffee. Perhaps you're enam-ored by her wisdom, care, and sensitivity. Or maybe you've felt sorry for her as you've commiserated together over her insensitive, brutish husband. You've held her as she cried. If so, you were lurking at your neighbor's door.

---

4. Why is the mind more difficult to control than the eyes? How will your eyes work together with your mind in your pursuit of sexual purity?
5. What do the authors mean by "lurking at the door" and "mental lurking"? What is your own experience with this?

Every Man's Walk
(Your Guide to Personal Application)

According to Jesus, doing it mentally is the same as doing it physically (see Matthew 5:28).

Currently, your mind runs like a mustang. What's more, your mind "mates" where it wills with attractive, sensual women. They're everywhere. With a mustang mind, how do you stop the running and the mating? With a corral around your mind.

_____

6. How seriously do you take Jesus's words in Matthew 5:28?

7. How would you explain the authors' corral concept as it applies to sexual purity in your thought life? What does the corral represent, and what does it accomplish?

8. How useful do you think this corral concept can be for you?

9. In quietness, review what you have written and learned in this week's study. If further thoughts or prayer requests come to your mind and heart, you may want to write them down.

Every Man's Talk
(Constructive Topics and Questions for Group Discussion)

Key Highlights from the Book for Reading Aloud and Discussing

_____

The defense perimeter of the mind is less like a wall and more like a customs area in an international airport. Customs departments are filters, preventing dangerous elements from entering a country. The defense perimeter of the mind works in a similar way by properly processing attractive women into your "country" while filtering out the alien seeds of attraction before the impure thoughts are even generated. This perimeter stops the lurking.

Jake: "I knew that kiss would end my career at my church, but I couldn't help myself."

_____

Discussion Questions

A. Which parts of chapter 14 in *Every Man's Battle* were most helpful or encouraging to you and why?

B. How would you explain the process, as explained in this chapter, by which the mind cleans away old sexual pollution? What encouragement does understanding this process give you?

C. What do the authors mean by a "mental customs station"? Describe this process in practical terms.

D. What do the authors mean by "starving the attractions"? What would it mean practically in your life?

E. Recall Fred's story of his high school crush on Judy—and the disaster prom date that ended it. Fred said, "My attractions to Judy died that night. The ugly facts . . . did them in!" Discuss the problem of filling in the blanks versus letting the facts do their attraction-reducing work.

> Note: If you're following a twelve-week track, save the rest of this lesson for the following week. If you're on the eight-week track, then keep going.

Every Man's Choice
(Questions for Personal Reflection and Examination)

There are two types of women who will approach your corral:

- Women who you find attractive
- Women who find you attractive

Both categories require similar defenses, and each is designed to starve the attractions until the women trot off toward the horizon again.

10. What are the most important principles for having effective defenses against impure thoughts regarding women you find attractive?

11. What are the most important principles for having effective defenses against impure thoughts regarding women who find you attractive?

12. What is your level of temptation *toward* old girlfriends and/or ex-wives? Wives of friends? What are the authors' most helpful suggestions to you in these areas?

Every Man's Walk
(Your Guide to Personal Application)

_____

Always play the dweeb. Players flirt; learn to unflirt. Players banter; learn to unbanter. If a woman smiles with a knowing look, learn to smile with a slightly confused look, to unsmile. If she talks about things that are hip, talk about things that are unhip to her, like your wife and kids. She'll find you pleasant enough but rather bland and uninteresting. *Perfect.*

It's not that you don't trust your friend's wife; it's that you don't want to start anything. She should be like a sister to you, with no hint of attraction between you.

You'll always have some relationship with your friend's wife, but limit it to when your friend is around. This isn't always possible, but these simple rules can shield you from surprise attacks within the corral.

_____

13. What do the authors mean by "playing the dweeb," and how effective do you think this tactic can be for you?

14. Review the four "shields" from surprise attacks related to friends' wives. Consider the practicality of each suggestion for your own life.

15. From the authors' entire strategy for purity—bouncing, starving, corralling, playing the dweeb, and so on—what is most important to ensure success in your own life?

16. a. What for you was the most meaningful concept or truth in this week's study?

   b. How would you talk this over with God? Write your response down as a prayer to Him.

   c. What do you believe God wants you to do in response to this week's study?

Every Man's Talk
(Constructive Topics and Questions for Group Discussion)

Key Highlights from the Book for Reading Aloud and Discussing

---

For those women who are already within your corral, the situation can become rather complicated. These women won't naturally drift back to the horizon once the attractions dissipate. They're in your corral today and probably will be there tomorrow and the next day. This means you must eliminate these attractions in some other fashion.

Let's take a look at the two main categories of women within your corral:

• Old girlfriends and ex-wives
• Wives of your friends

Purifying your eyes and mind is more than a command—it's also a sacrifice. As you make that sacrifice, as you lay down your desires, your maturity in the Lord will grow and blessings will flow. Your spiritual life will experience new health, joy, and stability, and your marital life will blossom as you learn to sacrifice your own desires for hers.

Discussion Questions

F. Which parts of chapters 15 and 16 in *Every Man's Battle* were most helpful or encouraging to you and why?

G. What tactics were presented for maintaining pure thoughts in regard to old girlfriends and ex-wives? What is your opinion of their effectiveness?

H. What tactics were presented for maintaining pure thoughts in regard to the wives of your friends? Why is it important to think through this strategy? (Spend several minutes talking about the practical implications for your group.)

7

Victory in Your Heart

This week's reading assignment:
chapters 17–18 in *Every Man's Battle*

Let's now consider the third perimeter, that innermost perimeter of your heart. To build out this section of your defenses, you must be consumed with God's purposes to cherish your wife. . . .

If Christians were consumed by God's purposes, it would first be reflected in our marriages. But the rates of divorce, adultery, and marital dissatisfaction in the church reveal the true state of our hearts.

We've known very few men consumed by their marriages and fewer still consumed by purity, yet God expects you to be consumed by both. God's purpose for marriage is that it parallel Christ's intimate, sacrificial relationship with His church so that you might be one with your wife.

—from chapter 17 in *Every Man's Battle*

Every Man's Truth
(Your Personal Journey into God's Word)

As you begin this study, take some time to read and meditate on the following Bible passage, which has to do with the beauty of the bride—the bride of Christ and also your own bride. Keep in mind that for centuries, Song of Songs has often been viewed as an allegory of how Christ feels for His bride (all believers).

> How beautiful you are, my darling!
> Oh, how beautiful!
> Your eyes behind your veil are doves. . . .
> Your lips are like a scarlet ribbon;
> Your mouth is lovely. . . .
> You are altogether beautiful, my darling;
> there is no flaw in you. . . .
>
> You have stolen my heart, my sister, my bride;
> you have stolen my heart
> with one glance of your eyes. . . .
> How delightful is your love, my sister, my bride! . . .
>
> Your head crowns you like Mount Carmel.
> Your hair is like royal tapestry;
> the king is held captive by its tresses.
> How beautiful you are and how pleasing,
> my love, with your delights!
> (Song of Songs 4:1, 3, 7, 9–10; 7:5–6)

1. Do you sense Jesus's desire for you as part of His bride? In return, does your heart yearn for Him like this?
2. Because our marriage relationships should parallel Christ's relationship to the church, our feelings for our wives should parallel these passages. Can you be

content with the wife of your youth? (If she isn't all you'd hoped for, remember that God graced you with this ewe lamb.)

3. Can you make a commitment to cherish her today?

Every Man's Choice
(Questions for Personal Reflection and Examination)

Are you sacrificially cherishing your wife? Do you feel those emotions for your wife as expressed in those passages [from Song of Songs]? I will admit that I haven't always felt that way. . . .

What about you? Has your heart for your wife withered?

If so, you probably got there the same way I did: by stopping short of God's purposes for marriage. God's primary standard is to unconditionally and sacrificially cherish her, no matter what. No conditions. But in America, we've mixed in our own ideas and diluted His standard, adding new, mealymouthed terms to create conditional contracts. . . .

Whenever we set conditions like these, we fix our gazes on what we expect to get from marriage for ourselves as the primary focus.

4. Review carefully the teaching in Ephesians 5:25–33 in light of all you've learned in this book and your study during the previous weeks. Why do you think so many husbands tend to resist the teaching of this passage?

5. State in your own words what the passage from Song of Songs teaches in regard to your marriage and Christ's relationship to the church. What are the right attitudes and convictions as taught in this passage? What are the right standards and ideals? What are the right actions and habits?

6. What does it really mean to you to cherish your wife?

7. What contractual conditions have you been trying to hold your wife to over the years? Were you consciously aware of doing this? What now needs to change?

Every Man's Walk
(Your Guide to Personal Application)

Your wife gave up her freedom for you. She relinquished her rights to seek happiness elsewhere. She exchanged this freedom for something she considered more valuable: your love and your word. Her dreams are tied up in you, dreams of sharing and communication and oneness.

She's pledged to be yours sexually. Her sexuality is her most guarded possession, her secret garden. She trusted you would be worthy of this gift, but you've regularly and cavalierly viewed sensual garbage, polluting and littering her garden. She deserves more, and you must honor that.

In my office, I keep an eight-by-ten black-and-white photo of Brenda from when she was a year old. Her little eyes sparkle and are filled with the hope and joy of life, her mischievous smile apparent even then with her glowing, chubby cheeks radiating joy and a carefree spirit. That face is so full of expectation and wonder. I brought that infant picture to my office because it reminds me that I need to honor that hope.

---

8. What has your wife given up for you? What are the most important things your wife has given to you?

9. What are the most important honor issues in your marriage? What are the most important ways you can build up and honor your wife's hope?

10. What can you do today to more faithfully honor your wife? What can you do tomorrow? What can you do as a new habit for the rest of your lives together?

11. In quietness, review what you have written and learned in this week's study. If further thoughts or prayer requests come to your mind and heart, you may want to write them down.

12. a. What for you was the most meaningful concept or truth in this week's study?

b. How would you talk this over with God? Write your response down as a prayer to Him.

c. What do you believe God wants you to do in response to this week's study?

Every Man's Talk
(Constructive Topics and Questions for Group Discussion)

Key Highlights from the Book for Reading Aloud and Discussing

---

How does matching Christ's relationship to His church help you build the inner perimeter and defend your sexual purity? The answer begins in your heart, where you may have selfish attitudes and expectations of your wife in marriage. When she doesn't meet these expectations, you become grumpy and frustrated and you pull away from her in your heart: *Well, if this is how she's going to be, why should I go through all the effort of being pure? She doesn't deserve it.*

So you retaliate by withdrawing your heart and pulling away from your responsibilities to love and cherish her.

Uriah knew his place. He was satisfied to fill his role in God's purposes.

If we're to be like Uriah, we must know our place and be content with it.

In our society, we have sensitivity training and cultural-enrichment classes. We believe that if we can only teach people the "right" feelings, they'll act correctly. In the Bible, however, God tells us the opposite: we're first to act correctly, and then right feelings will follow.

If you don't feel like cherishing, cherish anyway. Your right feelings will arrive soon enough.

A. Which parts of chapters 17 and 18 in *Every Man's Battle* were most helpful or encouraging to you and why?

B. When have you been grumpy and frustrated when your expectations for your wife haven't been met? Consider sharing about a recent example. How do you typically retaliate for unmet expectations?

C. Under the heading "Christ's Example" in chapter 17, look at the passages from Song of Songs. How would you analyze the feelings conveyed in these passages? How helpful are these passages as tools for understanding your proper emotional involvement with your wife?

D. Look at the quotation on the previous page about Uriah, and then review the story of David, Bathsheba, Uriah, and Nathan (from 2 Samuel 11–12) as summarized by the authors. This is probably a story you've read before. As you consider it again, what stands out to you now that you've carefully studied sexual purity and made a commitment to pursue it? What are the most important lessons this story has for Christian men today in their marriages?

E. Do you agree that we're to first act correctly and then right feelings will follow? Why or why not? What is your evidence?

8

Restoring Your Sexuality Together

This week's reading assignment:
chapters 19–20 in *Every Man's Battle*

Blocking out visual sensuality and unlearning that path to intensity is really what this book is all about. You've already studied how to get your eyes under control, and those defense perimeters impose deep and widespread synaptic changes in your brain. As you take these steps to bounce and starve your eyes, a subconscious wave of synaptic healing unfolds quite naturally, all without further effort from you.

—from chapter 20 in *Every Man's Battle*

Every Man's Truth
(Your Personal Journey into God's Word)

As you begin this study, take some time to read and meditate on the following Bible passage, which describes so beautifully the value of focusing all your attention on the wife God has blessed you with.

Let your fountain (wife) be blessed [with the rewards of fidelity],
And rejoice in the wife of your youth.

Let her be as a loving hind and graceful doe,
Let her breasts refresh and satisfy you at all times;
Always be exhilarated and delight in her love.

Why should you, my son, be exhilarated with an immoral woman
And embrace the bosom of an outsider (pagan)?

For the ways of man are directly before the eyes of the LORD,
And He carefully watches all of his paths [all of his comings and goings].

The iniquities done by a wicked man will trap him,
And he will be held with the cords of his sin.

He will die for lack of instruction (discipline),
And in the greatness of his foolishness he will go astray and be lost.
    (Proverbs 5:18–23, AMP)

1. Considering all we have learned in this book and study, why is it so important for a man to keep his focus on his wife?
2. What are the spiritual benefits and rewards of total fidelity to "the wife of your youth"?
3. On the other side, what do these verses from Proverbs reveal as the cost of being unfaithful with your eyes or lusting after a woman who is not your wife?
4. List some ideas of how you might better "rejoice in the wife of your youth"?

Every Man's Choice
(Questions for Personal Reflection and Examination)

Most in our culture remain at a disadvantage because they've been hood-winked by Hefner and others of his ilk who mainstreamed pornography and decoupled sex from a committed, marital relationship. They passed it off as sexual liberation and declared mission accomplished in their march on our sexuality and our society, which they proclaimed now free from the constraints of our Victorian past.

Today's raunchier, misogynistic porn, now delivered by an unprecedented access to streaming video, can so degrade a guy's neural sexual pathways that we have an epidemic of erectile dysfunction among men of all ages, even for those in their twenties and thirties.

5. What negative influences on your life have you experienced as a result of the mainstreaming of pornography by Hefner's *Playboy* magazine and similar media?

6. What temptations are you experiencing now from all the sources of pornography?

7. What tactics are you using to protect yourself from exposure—even accidental exposure—to pornography delivered on all your electronic devices?

Every Man's Walk
(Your Guide to Personal Application)

God perfectly grasps the addictive nature of that appetitive pleasure system with its all-in focus on intensity, but He wants something deeper and better for you: a soul connection that you may not have yet experienced in your life together, even after years of marriage.

8. What would be the qualities of an intimate soul connection between a husband and wife?

9. Do you believe you have such a connection with your wife? Why or why not?

10. What will be the advantages of a strong soul connection with your wife when you enter the latter years of your life?

Every Man's Talk
(Constructive Topics and Questions for Group Discussion)

Key Highlights from the Book for Reading Aloud and Discussing

_____

There is nothing wrong with outer beauty, but it shouldn't dominate our sexuality, and neither should our eyes, especially since the plasticity of our brain allows our tastes to flex and mold to our wife, if we'll only set our heart to let it happen. God has commanded you to always be ravished by the wife of your youth, but that is not possible if you keep lusting over buxom young babes.

It was my first experience with the paradox of obedience: the physically gratifying payoff resulting from obedience to God's sexual standards. . . . I actually got more intimate satisfaction from slowing down and cutting things back with Brenda. A kiss was no longer a joyless prerequisite on the path to intercourse; a kiss had become thrilling again.

If you rejoice only in the wife of your youth, and if you let only her breasts satisfy your eyes over the years, your sexual tastes will literally evolve and change along with her aging body. That capacity is already built into you as a man, which means that your obedience today will *enable* you to be exhilarated by your wife in the future, without effort and without a forceful act of your will. It will naturally unfold out of your makeup as a man.

If you *stop* lusting . . . , God has something better waiting for you: a wonderful partner you can grow old with and who can continue to satisfy you, even into the golden years. If you allow your tastes to change by walking in His truth and staying disciplined with your eyes, you will be ravished by the wife of your youth until the end of your lives.

_____

Discussion Questions

A. Which parts of chapters 19 and 20 in *Every Man's Battle* were most helpful or encouraging to you and why?

B. What have you learned in this study about the plasticity of the brain that can help you in winning the battle for sexual purity?

C. How would you describe true sexual liberation in terms of how God intended it to be?

D. The book describes the paradox of obedience as the physically gratifying payoff that comes from obedience to God's sexual standards. Why is such obedience a paradox or counterintuitive in today's "liberated" sexual culture?

E. Even though sex with your mate can be exciting and satisfying, what about such physical intimacy is also challenging for us men?

F. In your own words, describe what Fred meant when he wrote, "You're supposed to be having sex with the wonderful human soul *inside* your wife's tent."

G. Right now—and as you get older—how can you continue to improve in rejoicing "in the wife of your youth"?

H. Take a moment to reflect on what you've studied and discussed during the previous weeks. Comment on one or more of these questions: (1) What can you thank God for as a result of this study? (2) What do you sense that God most wants you to understand at this time about this topic? (3) In what specific ways do you believe He wants you to more fully trust and obey Him?

About the Authors

Stephen Arterburn is the founder and chairman of New Life Ministries, host of the daily *New Life Live!* national radio program, creator of the Women of Faith Conferences, and the author or coauthor of more than one hundred books with over eleven million in print. A nationally known speaker, Steve is also the editor of the best-selling *Life Recovery Bible* and *Every Man's Bible*. He has won numerous awards, including three Gold Medallions for writing excellence. In addition to attending seminary, he carries degrees from Baylor University and the University of North Texas, as well as two honorary doctorates, one from the California Graduate School of Theology. Steve resides with his family in Indiana, where he serves as the teaching pastor of Northview Church Carmel.

Fred Stoeker is the founder and president of Living True Ministries as well as a lay minister and popular conference speaker who travels internationally, challenging men to become sexually pure, to reconnect in true intimate relationships with their wives, and to train their sons to become godly men. Fred has counseled hundreds of married couples. In addition to being the coauthor of the best-selling Every Man series, he has written several books, including *Tactics* and *Hero*. Fred and his wife, Brenda, have written two books together, including the ECPA Silver Medallion winner *Every Heart Restored*. They live in the Des Moines, Iowa, area.

Mike Yorkey, a writer living in Encinitas, California, has collaborated with Fred Stoeker on all his books for the Every Man series.

To contact Steve or Fred about coaching, counseling, and speaking, please email:

sarterburn@newlife.com

fred@fredstoeker.com

EVERYMAN'S BATTLE
WORKSHOP

Winning the War on Sexual Temptation

Are you being controlled by lust, porn, affairs or a secret life? Are you afraid of being found out? Are you ready to live a life of freedom?

There is hope! The **Every Man's Battle Workshop** is an intensive 3-day **NO-SHAME zone** for men who want to have sexual integrity.

It doesn't matter what you've done. It doesn't matter where you've been. What matters is what you are willing to do now and what you will choose to do.

- Main sessions cover topics such as the nature of sexual temptation, false intimacy, restoring trust, and communication in marriage
- Small group sessions are led by counselors who have worked through their own sexual integrity issues

Join the millions across the country who have reclaimed their integrity, their faith, and are living in freedom.

Register Today!

For more information or to register,

call 800-NEW-LIFE (639-5433)

or go to NEWLIFE.COM

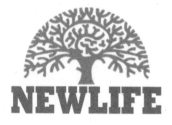

NEWLIFE

RESTORE

HOPE FOR A WOMAN'S HEART

Healing from the Pain of Betrayal

When you have suffered the pain of betrayal, you may feel overwhelmed, alone, angry and confused. Where can you find clarity on what to do? Who can help you along this journey you didn't plan to take?

At the **Restore Workshop** hope and healing as you journey together with other women who are exactly where you are.

Discover that restoration is possible—if not for your marriage, definitely for you. Find the tools you need to rebuild your future!

- Main sessions cover topics such as understanding addiction and the brain, anger, shame, and rebuilding trust
- Small group sessions are led by counselors who have worked through their own pain of betrayal

Find hope, develop connections, and discover a path towards restoration and wholeness!

Register Today!

For more information or to register, call 800-NEW-LIFE (639-5433) or go to NEWLIFE.COM

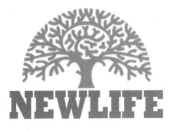

NEWLIFE